Outcome Measures in Home Care

Volume II
Service

Lynn T. Rinke, MS, RN, and Alexis A. Wilson, MPH, RN, Editors

Division of Accreditation for Home Care
and Community Health
National League for Nursing

Pub. No. 21-2195

National League for Nursing • New York

10-9-91

Manufactured in the United States of America.

CONTENTS

PREFACE

Home Care Outcomes: Focus on Practice

Access, cost, and quality are the principal motives shaping the public policy health agenda. In the mid-1960s, the political response to improving access to health care yielded the creation of Medicare and Medicaid. A decade later, cost-containment concerns drove health policy development, culminating with the introduction of the Medicare prospective payment system for hospital care. Now into the third decade of the nation's experiment with publicly financed health care, quality is assuming center stage on the health policy forum.

Issues surrounding quality assurance in health care delivery systems have run a course paralleling the evolution of health policy concerns. Although Donabedian introduced a comprehensive "structure-process-outcome" schema more than 20 years ago,[1] it is only now, in the late 1980s, that outcomes are receiving significant attention. Understandably, the maturing of quality assurance efforts mirrored public policy development. When federal initiatives focused on "access," the structural components of the health care system received great attention: Were there enough hospitals, nurses, doctors, mental health clinics, and so forth? As the federal perspective moved to examining ways to cut costs in health care delivery, the process components of quality became the focus of inquiry: What was the most efficient method of providing services? Was midwifery service comparable to obstetrical care? Could an outpatient clinic deliver comparable surgical services?

Now, having been preoccupied with access and cost, having explored and compared structural and process components, we are confronting the issue of quality head on. Ignited by concerns raised by the introduction of the Medicare prospective payment system, quality issues are directing policy development. In the practice sector, the ultimate response to the question of quality is to examine the outcomes of health care. For, as Donabedian (1974) stated, "The evolution of outcome is particularly attractive because it satisfies the eminently reasonable argument that all the health care in the world is for naught unless it makes some impact on health."[2]

Although it has taken some 20-plus years for the institutional and medical communities to seriously address outcome indicators of health care, the nursing profession has been grappling with this challenge since Florence Nightingale visited the Crimea. In particular, community health practitioners have been sensitive to the need to demonstrate the impact of their services on the health of their clients.

MEASURING THE OUTCOMES OF SERVICE

This volume presents a critical sample of efforts, both published and unpublished, to develop and measure outcome indicators for community-based nursing services. The pieces selected for inclusion represent a variety of perspectives on the question of what constitute pragmatic, useful outcomes against which to judge the quality of care delivered. The articles and examples also reflect a wide range of sophistication in both theoretical and applied science approaches. This diversity in perspective and sophistication is a conscious effort to reflect the realities of the community health practice community.

This anthology is the second in a new series of publications from the National League for Nursing focusing on community-based health services. Volume I of *Outcome Measures in Home Care* presents the important research on home care outcomes and addresses basic issues in evaluating quality. In publishing this series, we aim to contribute a broad resource for the work of the academic and practice communities in developing outcome-oriented quality assurance measures.

Part 1 presents a brief historical overview of the home care community's experience in outcome-based quality assurance efforts. Included are excerpts from the ANA's *Guidelines for Review of Nursing Care at the Local Level,* a classic primer on writing outcome standards; a descriptive report of the state of the art in 1979 by Flynn and Ray; and excerpts from another critical examination of the state of the art prepared by the American Bar Association in 1986.

Part 2 offers examples of promulgated outcome standards—standards developed by professional organizations for voluntary adoption by the practice community. These types of standards tend to be idealistic in nature, but provide direction and a framework for policy development as well as efforts to develop standards in individual organizations.

Part 3 offers examples of programmatic approaches to developing outcome standards for community-based services. This aggregate, population-based outcome approach is promoted in the NLN Accreditation Program for Home Care and Community Health, and one of the pieces was included as part of an agency self-study reports for accreditation.

The medical diagnosis approach to defining individual outcome standards is the focus of Section 4. In Section 5, other discipline-specific outcome approaches are explored. The first few examples identify home care outcomes from the perspectives of allied health disciplines such as physical and occupational therapies, speech pathology, and social work. The balance of the section offers an overview of professional nursing's efforts to define the outcomes of community health services.

Finally, Part 6 samples efforts to develop outcomes based on a functional status paradigm. As suggested by the variety of populations addressed in the articles in this section (mental health, rehabilitation, traditional home health care) functional status indicators may offer a mutlidisciplinary mechanism for identifying health outcomes.

As this book goes to press, a multitude of studies addressing the outcome of home care are in process. We hope that our effort to provide a historical and multidisciplinary overview of outcome measures for quality in home care will stimulate more research on the topic. In particular, we encourage readers to contact authors and agencies included herein to explore research efforts in the practice setting to expand nursing's knowledge base and to document the impact of home care services on the health of the communities we serve.

—Lynn T. Rinke, MS, RN

REFERENCES

1. A. Donabedian, "Evaluating the Quality of Medical Care, *Milbank Memorial Fund Quarterly,* 44 (July 1966), Part 2, 166–206.
2. A. Donabedian, "Some Basic Issues in Evaluating the Quality of Health Care," *Issues in Evaluation Research* (Kansas City, MO: American Nurses' Association, 1976), 3–28. Reprinted in L. T. Rinke, ed., *Outcome Measures in Home Care, Vol. I* (New York: National League for Nursing, 1987), 3–28.

Part 1

History and Overview

Guidelines for Review of Nursing Care at the Local Level

In response to 1972 legislation establishing the Professional Standards Review Organization system for evaluating the quality of health care, the American Nurses' Association published Guidelines for Review of Nursing Care at the Local Level. *This volume presents a comprehensive model for developing quality assurance criteria to assess nursing services in a multitude of settings. Excerpted here are sections addressing the development of outcome criteria, with examples applicable for posthospitalization outcomes. This particular model for developing standards was used by a number of agencies in the 1970s.*

DEVELOPING OUTCOME CRITERIA

Rationale for the Use of Outcome Criteria

The question of defining an acceptable level of care can be answered from the perspectives of structure, process, and outcome. In any review process a decision must be made whether structure, process, or outcome criteria are appropriate, or whether all three types of criteria or combinations are appropriate. The three types of criteria are interrelated. Structure influences process and outcome; process influences structure and outcome; outcomes

influence structure and process. All three perspectives of quality are important. It is often assumed that structure criteria, such as staffing ratio, lead
to effective health care. Another assumption may be that when nurses follow
a designated process a predictable change will occur in the patient. In other
words, instructing the patient (process) does not mean that the patient will
learn (outcome). However, such assumptions and expectations are not acceptable measures of quality of care or of a resulting change in health status.
The end result of care for a patient can only be documented by outcome.

> The evaluation of outcome is particularly attractive because it satisfies
> the eminently reasonable argument that all the health care in the world
> is for naught unless it makes some impact on health. Moreover, most
> people agree on what are desired health outcomes, so that the criteria
> enjoy a great deal of face validity. Finally, health outcomes have an in-
> tegrative property that seems to solve many of the problems of quality
> assessment. At the level of the individual patient, outcomes represent
> the result of the efforts of all those who have been involved in that pa-
> tient's care. At the population level, health outcomes represent the opera-
> tion of the health services system as a whole, including the effects of
> access, resource allocation, external benefits, and the conformity of pro-
> fessional performance to professional norms. Thus, we seem to have sum-
> marized in one measure all that we need to know.[1]

Maintaining the focus of the criteria on the state of the patient focuses
the attention of the practitioner on whether or not what he/she does makes
a difference to the patient. Outcome criteria allow for a wide variety of nursing interventions since these criteria ask only whether or not the interventions were effective. For example, achievement of the criterion, "patient has
intact skin," may require any or all effective nursing interventions related
to hygiene, safety, hydration, nutrition, and circulation. The use of outcome
criteria for screening large numbers of patients is not inconsistent with individualized care.

The use of outcome criteria to screen large numbers of patient populations is
of value for efficiency and economy of review. Most of the evaluation of nursing care has been based on process criteria. This requires trained observers and
interviewers and developing or using complex criteria covering a wide variety of
behaviors of each person involved in delivering the care to clients. However, for
the situations in which a retrospective review based on patient outcomes indicates a need to review the behavior of the nurse(s), there are several techniques
for process evaluation that have been carefully developed, tested, and published
which can be utilized for further evaluation of the quality of nursing care.

The use of outcome criteria is also practical for use in all clinical settings.
Within PSRO, outcome criteria will be used in medical (health) care evaluation studies to document the appropriateness, necessity, and effectiveness
of nursing care.

The Writers of Outcome Criteria

There is continuing controversy and debate about who should write out-come criteria. Should criteria be established by nurses, practitioners, ad-ministrators, or educators? Should criteria be established by nurses within hospitals or health agencies or should there be regional or national criteria? In this manual the position is taken that the practicing nurse in the local set-ting is in the best possible position to identify quality of nursing care and should participate in criteria development. Once developed, sets of outcome criteria should be shared so that costly duplication of effort can be avoided. Criteria developed at the national level can serve as examples to be considered by the nurse at the local level.

Groups of nurse peers can establish criteria to evaluate the care of pa-tients within their practice. Nurses with a patient load of intensive cardiac patients can establish the criteria for that patient population; maternity nurses can establish the criteria for primary maternity clients. These groups of nurses may give consideration to existing sets of criteria, then make the decision to accept the existing set, to modify an existing set, or to write their own.

Since those who write the criteria are not necessarily the ones who carry out the review, the importance of having clear and precise criteria cannot be overemphasized.

Guidelines for Developing Sets of Outcome Criteria Statements

The value of the entire review procedure lies in the quality of the criteria used for patient care review. The development of criteria needs to follow guidelines which will assure relevance and recognition by peers within the specific health care system.

The following guidelines may be helpful in developing outcome criteria:

1. Screening criteria are a crucial (critical) factor that, if not met, may indicate a significant deficiency in nursing.
2. The purpose of screening criteria is to survey a large number of cases and quickly determine acceptable levels of patient outcomes.
3. The outcome stated in criteria must be possible to achieve.
4. Criteria should be statements of specific outcomes representing op-timal achievement.
5. Criteria should be written as specifically as possible, including the time when it is to be measured and the measurement to be used to determine if the criteria have been met.

6. In establishing criteria, select the most critical time for the measurement of the identified outcome for a particular patient population.

7. Criteria must be appraisable. However, the ease of measurement should be used as the sole basis for accepting or rejecting potential criteria. If criteria are important, some assessment can usually be obtained.

8. Criteria should be stated to yield a dichotomous distinction (yes—no).

9. Criteria should be phrased in positive terms (presence of) rather than negative terms (absence of), when applicable.

10. Criteria should be pertinent to the particular patient population under consideration. For example, for the ambulatory patient receiving photocoagulation of the eye, skin care is not a priority. Hence, criteria would not be written for skin care.

11. Criteria should be free from bias. Each patient to whom criteria are applied should have an equal opportunity to meet the criteria. For example, skin condition for an aged patient and a youth might require different criteria.

12. A set of criteria applicable to a specific patient population may include criteria for outcomes of care for members of the family or significant others.

Establishing criteria is a "pencil and eraser" operation. Criteria will change as values and scientific knowledge change. Criteria are never considered final. As practice changes, criteria sets should be revised at regular intervals.

The Process of Writing Outcome Criteria

There is a natural flow of steps for writing outcome criteria:

- Choose a category.
- Identify the target population.
- Select the appropriate population variables.
- Select criteria subsets, if desired.
- Generate outcome criteria.
- Establish the critical time.
- Establish the standard.
- Establish any exceptions to the criteria and standards.
- Document the sources for the criteria.
- Choose preliminary selection of screening criteria.

Sample criteria that have been developed for a target population, respiratory distress, can be found in Figure 1. This sample is used as an illustration in the following description of the process of developing outcome criteria.

Choose a Category. Patient populations can be selected using any of the categories: nursing problem/diagnosis, medical diagnosis, developmental stages, syndromes/symptoms, body systems, concepts, e.g., rehabilitation.

As an example, an institution may wish to select patient population categories using a medical diagnosis in order to facilitate the retrieval of the charts. If the medical diagnosis is chosen, it may be necessary to identify the associated nursing problems or nursing diagnoses that are primarily influenced by nursing care. For example, with a patient category myocardial infarction/self-image change, nurses can affect the area of self-image change. Nurses cannot prescribe treatments or medications that will affect the heart itself.

Another example of a category that might be chosen is syndrome. Patient populations under this category could include the grief syndrome or rape trauma syndrome. In the example, respiratory distress, the patients are categorized according to a syndrome.

When identifying patient populations, use only a single category to define each population. Multiple problems within the same category should not be used in the first attempt to define the patient population under study. For example, do not use diabetes with a fractured femur. However, categories can be combined. Cardiovascular accident (a medical diagnosis) could be combined with immobility (nursing problem or diagnosis).

Identify the Target Population. The next major decision is the selection of a group of patients for whom criteria are to be developed. A patient population is defined as a group of people with like characteristics. Patients with the medical diagnosis of diabetes mellitus or with a nursing diagnosis of preoperative anxiety are examples of different patient populations that might be used.

The population should be selected based on local experience and practice. Patient populations must be representative of the persons served by nurses in a specific institution, agency, or practice. Begin by selecting the most common patient populations. In other words, select patients with encephalitis only if this type of patient is common to the practice.

Patient populations may be selected in cooperation with a multidisciplinary quality assurance committee or audit committee. If a record audit is the method for collecting data, it is economical to consider having the same data abstracting personnel and records used for several disciplines.

Patient populations should be selected in collaboration with medical records personnel if they are to retrieve data for collection or audit. Medical records

FIGURE 1
Sample Criteria for a Target Population

CRITERIA DEVELOPMENT WORKSHEET

TARGET POPULATION : Respiratory Distress

Maternal & Child Health Nursing
Task Force

These model criteria are for screening patient care for subsequent peer review and do not constitute standards of care governing a nurse's or agency's obligation to a patient.

Variables:

a. Hospitalized to 4 weeks post-hospital
b. Pneumonia and/or bronchitis
c. 1½ to 3 years old
d. No history of chronic illness/anomalies
e. No concurrent illness

PARENT: Term used to describe any individual fulfilling parenting role.

CRITERIA SUBSET	SCREENING CRITERIA	CRITICAL TIME	*STANDARD	EXCEPTION	DOCUMENTATION
Maintenance of adequate cardio-pulmonary function.	The patient will:				
	Sleep or rest for interval of at least ½ hour	4 hours	100%		Blake, F., Wright, F.H., and Waeckter, E., Nursing Care of Children, Philadelphia J.B. Lippincott Co., 1970, p. 244.
	Have pink mucous membranes in a controlled environment	2 hours	100%		Ibid.
	Have pink nailbeds in a con-trolled environment	2 hours	100%		Gellis and Kagan. Current Pediatric Therapy. Philadelphia: W.B. Saunders Co., 1970, p. 185.
	Have a rectal temperature less than 100° F within one hour after febrile episode	8 hours	100%		Blake, p. 244. Gellis and Kagan, p. 185.
	Have a respiratory rate be-tween 20-36/minute in a controlled environment	48 hours	100%		Ross Laboratories. Children are Different: Relation of Age to Physiologic Function, Columbus, Ohio: Ross Laboratories, 1970, p. 18.
	Be febrile without antipyretic agents	48 hours	100%		Wasserman, E., and L. Slobody. Survey of Clinical Pediatrics. New York: McGraw-Hill Book Co., 1974, pp. 352-56.
	Not require suctioning	Third day	100%		Blake, p. 247
	Have a respiratory rate be-tween 20-36/minute out of controlled environment	Fourth day	100%		Gellis and Kagan, pp. 179-80.
	Have thin secretions easily removed by suctioning	12 hours	100%		Ross Laboratories, p. 18.
	Have heart rate within normal limits: 90-120 BPM	48 hours	100%		Chinn, Peggy, and Cynthia Leitch. Child Health Maintenance. St. Louis: C.V. Mosby

FIG. 1 (continued)

CRITERIA DEVELOPMENT WORKSHEET

Population No. 7

TARGET POPULATION : Respiratory Distress

These model criteria are for screening patient care for subsequent peer review and do not constitute standards of care governing a nurse's or agency's obligation to a patient.

Variables:

a. Hospitalized to 4 weeks post-hospital
b. Pneumonia and/or bronchitis
c. 1½ to 3 years
d. No history of chronic illness/anomalies
e. No concurrent illness

PARENT : Term used to describe any individual fulfilling parenting role

CRITERIA SUBSET	SCREENING CRITERIA	CRITICAL TIME	*STANDARD	EXCEPTION	DOCUMENTATION
	The patient will: Have pink mucous membranes and nailbeds out of controlled environment	Fourth day	100%		
	Have chest clear on auscultation (no rales or ronchi)	Fifth day	100%		
Maintenance of adequate hydration and electrolyte balance	Have a total fluid intake for age cc/240 (see formula)	24 hours	100%		NOTE: (10 Kg) 85 cc/Kg, (15 Kg) 63 cc/Kg = 24 hour maintenance needs to cover sensible, insensible and urinary losses. Kempe, C. Henry, et al. *Current Pediatric Diagnosis and Treatment.* Los Altos, California: Lang Medical Publications, 1974, p. 923.
	Retain an adequate oral intake	Fourth day	100%		
	Void once	By 4 hours	100%		
	Void at least 4 times per day	24 hours	100%		
	Take and retain solid foods	Third day	100%		
	Have electrolytes within normal range: NA--136-143 meq/100cc	24 hours	100%		Ibid. pp. 987-992
	Potassium -- 4.1-5.6	24 hours	100%		
	Chloride -- 97-104	24 hours	100%		
	Carbon Dioxide -- 18-23	24 hours	100%		
Parent participates in management of child's illness	Parent will: Express (verbally or non-verbally) feelings about child's illness	Throughout hospitalization	100%		Blake. *Nursing Care of Children,* pp. 45-46.
	Hold or stay with, or talk with child during or after medical treatment	2 days	100%		Petrillo, M., and S. Sanger. *Emotional Care of Hospitalized Children.* Philadelphia: J.B. Lippincott Co., 1972, pp. 53-98.

*Chart Review Standard

FIG. 1 (continued)

CRITERIA DEVELOPMENT WORKSHEET

TARGET POPULATION: Respiratory Distress

Maternal & Child Health Nursing Task Force

These model criteria are for screening patient care for subsequent peer review and do not constitute standards of care governing a nurse's or agency's obligation to a patient.

Variables:
a. Hospitalized to 4 weeks post-hospital
b. Pneumonia and/or bronchitis
c. 1½ to 3 years
d. No history of chronic illness/anomalies
e. No concurrent illness

PARENT: Term used to describe any individual fulfilling parenting role

CRITERIA SUBSET	SCREENING CRITERIA	CRITICAL TIME	*STANDARD	EXCEPTION	DOCUMENTATION
	Parent will:				
	Participate in daily care activities by helping feed or helping bathe or toileting child	Second day	100%		Chinn and Leitch. *Child Health Maintenance.* p. 261.
	Actively participate in discharge plans by asking about discharge plans for taking child home, and talking about how she will manage at home	Second day	100%		Ibid.
	Parent prioritizes responsibilities to ill child and other family members	2 days	100%		Ibid.
Adaptation of child to hospitalization	Child will exhibit normal protesting behaviors of:				Blake. *Nursing Care of Children.* pp. 293-300.
	Cry, cling, fight or push substitute away when separated from parent	Throughout hospitalization	100%		Petrillo and Sanger. *Emotional Care of Hospitalized Children.* pp. 66-68, pp. 141-43.
	Cry, cling, fight, or push substitute away when faced with intrusive procedures, such as temperatures, injection, and suctioning	Throughout hospitalization	100%		*Attachment and Loss.* ed. J. Bowlby. vol. 2: *Separation.* New York: Basic Books, 1973, chapter 3.
	Child will relax extremities, talk and/or cuddle with other caring person within 10 minutes of separation from parent	Second day	100%		Chinn and Leitch, pp. 423-25.
Maintenance of child's preillness developmental level	Child will show behaviors of mastering his environment by:				
	Crawling or walking or feeding self, or talking or playing or potty behaviors	Fourth day	100%		Petrillo and Sanger, p. 143.
	Child shows interest in surroundings with staring, pointing, and reaching for objects in the surroundings	Second day	100%		Chinn and Leitch, pp. 207-25.

*Chart Review Standard

FIG. 1 (continued)

CRITERIA DEVELOPMENT WORKSHEET

TARGET POPULATION : Respiratory Distress

Maternal & Child Health Nursing
Task Force

Variables:
a. Hospitalized to 4 weeks post-hospital
b. Pneumonia and/or bronchitis
c. 1½ to 3 years
d. No history of chronic illness/anomalies
e. No concurrent illness

*These model criteria are for screen-
ing patient care for subsequent peer
review and do not constitute standards of care governing a nurse's
or agency's obligation to a patient.*

CRITERIA SUBSET	SCREENING CRITERIA	CRITICAL TIME	*STANDARD	EXCEPTION	DOCUMENTATION
Child's reentry into home/family unit	The child will:				
	Interact with parents in same level of attachment as preillness as validated by nurse with parent	4 weeks post discharge	100%		Chinn and Leitch. *Child Health Maintenance,* pp. 423-24.
	Resume preillness levels of sleep, play, eating, and elimination	4 weeks post discharge	100%		Blake. *Nursing Care of Children,* p. 35.
	The parent will:				Chinn and Leitch, p. 414.
	State symptoms of respiratory distress	Discharge	100%		
	State what to do if symptoms occur	Discharge	100%		
	Name each take-home medication	Discharge	100%		
	State side-effects of each medication	Discharge	100%		
	State correct dosage of each medication	Discharge	100%		
	State schedule for giving medications	Discharge	100%		
	State the need to keep the medication safe from the reach of her children	Discharge	100%		
	Return child to health care provider for followup care	Scheduled visit 1 week post discharge	100%		Petrillo and Sanger, pp. 83-84.
	Parents can describe potential and/or anticipated changes in child's behavior upon reentry into family unit	At discharge	100%		
	Parent prepares other family members for child's return home	Discharge	100%		

*Chart Review Standard

FIG. 1 (continued)

CRITERIA DEVELOPMENT WORKSHEET

Population No. 7

TARGET POPULATION : Respiratory Distress

Maternal & Child Health Nursing
Task Force

These model criteria are for screening patient care for subsequent peer review and do not constitute standards of care governing a nurse's or agency's obligation to a patient.

Variables:
a. Hospitalized to 4 weeks post-hospital
b. Pneumonia and/or bronchitis
c. 1½ to 3 years
d. No history of chronic illness/anomalies
e. No concurrent illness

CRITERIA SUBSET	SCREENING CRITERIA	CRITICAL TIME	*STANDARD	EXCEPTION	DOCUMENTATION
	Parent can describe nutrition: Basic four and their relationship to preventive health care	Discharge	100%		
	Parent is able to care for child at health level at discharge	Discharge	100%		

*Chart Review Standard

personnel can give valuable information about the number and kind of variables used for each population.

There should also be an established knowledge base for nursing intervention for the patient populaton. The patient population should be one that is influenced by nursing intervention as documented in the literature or by experts. *It is not necessary that the patient population be influenced exclusively by nursing. Most patients will be affected by several disciplines, but would be appropriate for nursing review if the nurse affects any alteration in the patient's status.*

Select appropriate population variables. Patient populations must be specific. They must be described by a well-defined set of variables or characteristics. Examples of variables may include:

Age	Genetic factors
Sex	Health history
Race	Disability index
Significant others	Cultural differences
Place of residence	Degree of illness
Living arrangements	Medical problem
Education	Nursing problem
Occupation	Risk factors
Income	Functional classification
Health financing	Degree of limitation
Travel distance	Religious orientation
Travel time	Availability of transportation
Referral source	Accessibility of health facilities

The number of variables should be large enough to identify a patient population with similar characteristics, yet small enough so that enough patients can be found that fit the characteristics. Select variables for which data are available and retrievable.

The general target population respiratory distress is too large a population to be studied. Too many variables exist within that general population to establish valid criteria for care. A number of variables have been selected to reduce the population being studied and to make the group more homogeneous. The variables in this example are:

- Hospitalized to four weeks posthospital.
- Pneumonia and/or bronchitis.
- 1½- to 3-year-old child.
- No history of chronic illness/anomalies.
- No concurrent illness.

These variables limit the group so that a number of criteria can be identified for these patients to indicate whether or not they are receiving adequate care.

Select criteria subsets. Oftentimes groups developing criteria may find it helpful to organize criteria for patient populations into subsets (headings) based on categories of nursing concern. Criteria subsets might be determined by nursing diagnosis, nursing problems, nursing concerns, functional problems, functional states, nursing theories, and developmental states. Criteria subsets should provide an organizational framework. Criteria subsets are not necessary for generating outcome criteria, but they may be useful to organizing the development of criteria and to assure that all aspects of patient care—biological, psychological, and sociocultural—have been covered in a list of outcome criteria.

In the example, general criteria subsets used to organize the criteria for the respiratory distress target population include biological, psychological, and social factors:

Maintenance of adequate cardiopulmonary function (biological).

Maintenance of adequate hydration and electrolyte balance (biological).

Parent participates in management of child's illness (psychological).

Adaptation of child to hospitalization (social).

Maintenance of child's pre-illness developmental level (psychological).

Child's reentry into home/family unit (psychosocial).

Generate Outcome Criteria. All suggestions should be recorded when generating the first list of criteria. (The nominal group process has been found to be effective in generating these suggestions.) The list is examined for duplication or omissions. These suggestions are then revised to assure that they are written in measurable terms. Each is then termed a criterion statement. If the purpose of the review is to develop a set of comprehensive criteria, then all criteria may be retained. If the purpose is to develop a set of screening criteria, the selection process would be limited to a few very important criteria. The outcome criteria listed in the respiratory distress example are comprehensive in nature.

Establish Critical Times. Criteria should have some kind of time limitation. A time needs to be established within which that criterion will be met. A commonly used critical time is the time of discharge, however, other critical times might be upon admission, upon discharge from recovery area, upon discharge from intensive care unit, 24 hours after surgery, three months after admission to a nursing home, one year after care identification in a public health agency, eight hours after admission.

The question to be answered is, "By what time in the progress of the patient's care should these criteria be met?'' In the respiratory distress example, the criterion states, "The patient will sleep or rest for an interval of at least one-half hour." A critical time of four hours has been chosen, the result being that this criterion will be met only if the individual patient rests for one-half hour within four hours of admission.

Establish the Standard. The recommended standard to be used for screening purposes is 100 percent. Criteria should be achieved 100 percent of the time or by 100 percent of the patients. By setting this standard, all cases not meeting this level must be examined and a reason determined for the lack of achievement. The standard established for screening purposes may be different than the standard of an acceptable practice established for the group of patients, providers, or units. The 100 percent screening standard assures that all charts not meeting the criteria will "fall through" the screen and thus can be reviewed in detail. After a review of the "unacceptable" charts, it may be decided that a 75 percent compliance standard is acceptable considering the circumstances of the particular setting. As more data are examined, it may be feasible to modify the screening standard or to modify the criteria.

Establish Exceptions to the Criteria. Exceptions to the criteria should be noted at this point. This column should not have many entries. It may be unrealistic to expect a person having emergency surgery to demonstrate coughing and deep breathing exercises prior to surgery; therefore, emergency surgery may be listed as an exception. Language barriers, mental retardation, and other preexisting problems may also be exceptions.

Document the Sources for the Criteria. The most frequent source will be the literature. The results of nursing research should be incorporated into the sets of outcome criteria when available.

Preliminary Selection of Screening Criteria. The writers of the comprehensive sets of criteria will undoubtedly want a limited number or a set of screening criteria by which large populations can be reviewed.

REVISION AND VALIDATION OF SCREENING CRITERIA SETS

Revising and validating criteria are continuous processes. There must be a built-in mechanism of communication among practitioners to develop a sense of involvement. After the critical criteria have been identified, the first step is to make certain that the guidelines for criteria development have been met.

Before criteria are put to any test, they should also be editorially revised. When it is possible, the people who wrote the criteria should not be involved in revising them. These individuals, however, should be given an opportunity to react to the revisions prior to an audit.

The following points may be helpful when doing an editorial revision:

1. Arrange criteria in chronological order from the time of patient's admission or initial contact to patient's discharge and after.

2. Arrange criteria, when possible, by their location in the client's record; e.g., blood pressure, pulse, respiration, and temperature are located together in the chart.

3. Arrange criteria under similar headings to shorten the form and provide ease in reading.

4. Reword criteria if necessary to state the outcome desired, *not* the process which was followed to produce the outcome.

5. Include only one criterion for each outcome. If there are two criteria dealing with the same outcome, eliminate one.

6. Use a consistent format in writing critical times; e.g., "by the end of" is a statement which can be used for all critical times pertaining to a population. Other examples might include "48 hours after surgery," "by the end of the first day," or "throughout hospitalization."

7. Eliminate all abbreviations except accepted medical abbreviations.

8. Eliminate examples unless absolutely essential to interpret the criteria.

9. Use action verbs in the same tense; eliminate abstract verbs.

10. Be sure criteria are written in observable terms to minimize individual interpretations.

11. Indicate the person expected to perform the outcome, e.g., patient, significant others, family, etc.

12. Criteria should contain only one idea.

13. Eliminate ambiguous terms such as "good" or "well."

14. Write criteria as expected outcomes for a group of patients from the same population rather than for an individual patient.

15. Eliminate criteria which are not exclusive or significant indicators of nursing care.

16. Eliminate criteria that are not considered screening criteria (absolutely essential to measure acceptable nursing care).

A second step in revising and validating criteria might be agreement testing, or ratification of the criteria (cross validation). This requires some means of determining how many nurses agree on the criteria. A set of criteria written by one group of nurses can be given to another group of peer nurses who are then asked to rate the criteria as to whether or not the criteria are appropriate indicators of nursing care for that population. By rating the criteria on a Likert-type scale, these reviewing nurses act as judges. They use their professional judgment and clinical experience in making these decisions. The judges may also be asked to indicate their rationale for rating any criteria neutral, disagree, or strongly disagree. Suggestions for revisions of criteria can also be elicited. A sample format for agreement testing is illustrated in Figure 2. Criteria which have been edited for the target population—respiratory distress—are included.

Reliability and Validity Studies

Criteria development can also be tested to determine (a) whether or not the measurement is consistent, and (b) whether or not the criteria reflect quality nursing care. In other words, criteria need to be tested for reliability and validity. Although some research studies in the area of reliability and validity are currently underway, many more need to be undertaken.[2]

USE OF THE CRITERIA

Using the criteria completes the Model for Quality Assurance described in Chapter 2 of this manual. The initial use of outcome criteria would be as a screen for the quality of care provided for a large number of patients. An example of a retrospective chart audit form for the respiratory distress example is given in Figure 3. The actual procedure will, in most institutions, be performed by medical records personnel.

A summary of the audit finding will be returned to the review committee for decisions on courses of action indicated by the data. Clinical settings beginning audits frequently encounter insufficient data upon which to evaluate the care. In such cases, courses of action to improve documentation are indicated. Sharing the results of the audit and reviewing the criteria upon which it was based may be sufficient motivation for more relevant charting. Additional actions may include a series of educational sessions on problem-oriented recording or the legal aspects of charting. Regardless of the choice, a measurement of change in the processes or structure of charting should be made and the same criteria upon which action was based should be used in the follow-up audit. One decision may be that the criteria are not critical indicators of care. A return to the beginning of this criteria-writing

FIGURE 2
Sample Format for Testing Agreement of Criteria

SCREENING CRITERIA FOR TARGET POPULATION

RESPIRATORY DISTRESS: HOSPITALIZED
Pneumonia and/or Bronchitis
1½ to 3 Years; No History of Chronic Illness/Anomalies
No Concurrent Illness

Remember you are to indicate the degree to which you feel the criteria below indicate an acceptable level of nursing care for the above population.

SCREENING CRITERIA	STRONGLY DISAGREE	DISAGREE	NEUTRAL OR UNDECIDED	AGREE	STRONGLY AGREE	REASON(S) FOR RATING	SUGGESTION(S)
THROUGHOUT HOSPITALIZATION, the PARENT							
1. expressed verbally or nonverbally feelings about the child's illness.							
THROUGHOUT HOSPITALIZATION, the CHILD exhibited protesting behaviors (e.g., cried, clung, fought, or pushed substitute away) when							
2. separated from parent							
3. faced with intrusive procedures (e.g., temperatures, injections, suctioning).							
TWO HOURS after hospitalization, the PATIENT had							
4. pink mucous membranes in a controlled environment							
5. pink nailbeds in a controlled environment.							
FOUR HOURS after hospitalization, the PATIENT							
6. slept or rested for intervals of at least ½ hour							
7. voided once.							
EIGHT HOURS after hospitalization if the PATIENT had a febrile spike							
8. within one hour the rectal temperature was less than 100° F.							
TWENTY-FOUR HOURS after hospitaliziationt the PATIENT							
9. had a total fluid intake for age cc/24 hr. [as determined by (10Kg) (85 cc/kg), (15kg) 63 cc/kg) = 24 hr. maintenance needs].							
10. voided at least 4 times.							
FORTY-EIGHT HOURS after hospitalization the PATIENT							
11. had a respiratory rate between 20-36/minute in controlled environment							

FIG. 2 (continued)

RESPIRATORY DISTRESS: HOSPITALIZED
Pneumonia and/or Bronchitis
1½ to 3 Years; No History of Chronic Illness/Anomalies
No Concurrent Illness

SCREENING CRITERIA	STRONGLY DISAGREE	DISAGREE	NEUTRAL OR UNDECIDED	AGREE	STRONGLY AGREE	REASON(S) FOR RATING	SUGGESTION(S)
12. was afebrile without antipyretic agents							
13. relaxed extremities, talked, and/or cuddled with other caring person within 10 minutes of separation from parent.							
FORTY-EIGHT HOURS after hospitalization the PARENT							
14. held, stayed with, or talked with child during or after medical treatment							
15. participated in daily care activities (e.g., helping to feed, bathe, or toilet child)							
16. actively participated in discharge plans (e.g., asks about discharge, states plans for taking child home, and talks about how she will manage at home).							
THREE DAYS after hospitalization, the PATIENT							
17. did not require suctioning.							
FOUR DAYS after hospitalization the PATIENT							
18. had a respiratory rate between 20-36/minute out of controlled environment							
19. retained an adequate oral intake [(10Kg) (85cc/Kg), (15Kg) 63cc/Kg – 24 hour maintenance needs]							
20. demonstrated behaviors of mastering his environment (e.g., crawling, walking, feeding self, talking, playing, or potty behaviors).							
At time of DISCHARGE, the PARENT							
21. stated symptoms of respiratory distress							
22. stated what to do if symptoms occur							
23. named each take-home medication							
24. stated side-effects of each medication							
25. stated correct dosage of each medication							
26. stated schedule for giving medications							
27. stated the need to keep the medication safe from the reach of her children.							

****
* *
* These model criteria are for screen- *
* ing patient care for subsequent peer *
* review and do not constitute stan- *
* dards of care governing a nurse's *
* or agency's obligation to a patient. *
* *
****

FIGURE 3
Example of Retrospective Chart Audit Form

SCREENING CRITERIA FOR TARGET POPULATION
RESPIRATORY DISTRESS:
Hospitalized; Pneumonia and/or Bronchitis
1½ to 3 Years; No History of Chronic Illness/Anomalies
No Concurrent Illness

SCREENING CRITERIA	CLEARLY CHARTED MET	CLEARLY CHARTED NOT MET	INSUFFICIENT DATA FOR DECISION	SOURCE OF CRITERIA
TWO HOURS after hospitalization the PATIENT had				
1. pink mucous membranes in a controlled environment				
2. pink nailbeds in a controlled environment				
FOUR HOURS after hospitalization the PATIENT				
3. slept or rested for intervals of at least ½ hour				
4. voided once				
TWENTY-FOUR HOURS after hospitalization the PATIENT				
5. had a total fluid intake for age cc/24 hr. [as determined by (10 Kg) 85 cc/Kg, (15 Kg) 63 cc/Kg = 24 hr. maintenance needs]				
6. voided at least 4 times				
FORTY-EIGHT HOURS after hospitalization the PATIENT				
7. had a respiratory rate between 20-36/minute in controlled environment				
8. was afebrile without antipyretic agents				
9. relaxed extremities, talked, and/or cuddled with other caring person within 10 minutes of separation from parent				
10. exhibited protesting behaviors (e.g., cried, clung, fought, or pushed substitute away) when				
a. separated from parent				
b. faced with intrusive procedures (e.g., temperatures, injections, suctioning)				
FORTY-EIGHT HOURS after hospitalization the PARENT				
11. expressed verbally or nonverbally feelings about child's illness				
12. held, stayed with, or talked with child during or after medical treatment				
13. participated in daily care activities (e.g., helping to feed, bathe, or toilet child)				
These model criteria are for screening patient care for subsequent peer review and do not constitute standards of care governing a nurse's or agency's obligation to a patient.				

FIG. 3 (continued)

RESPIRATORY DISTRESS:
Hospitalized; Pneumonia and/or Bronchitis
1½ to 3 Years; No History of Chronic Illness/Anomalies
No Concurrent Illness

SCREENING CRITERIA	CLEARLY CHARTED MET	CLEARLY CHARTED NOT MET	INSUFFICIENT DATA FOR DECISION	SOURCE OF CRITERIA
14. actively participated in discharge plans (e.g., asks about discharge, states plans for taking child home, and talks about how she will manage at home)				
FOUR DAYS after hospitalization the PATIENT				
15. had a respiratory rate between 20-36/ minute out of controlled environment				
16. retained an adequate oral intake [(10 Kg) (85 cc/Kg),(15 Kg) 63 cc/Kg = 24 hour needs]				
17. demonstrated behaviors of mastering his environment (e.g., crawling, walking, feeding self, talking, playing, or potty behaviors)				
At time of DISCHARGE, the PARENT				
18. stated symptoms of respiratory distress				
19. stated what to do if symptoms occur				
20. named each take-home medication				
21. stated side-effects of each medication				
22. stated correct dosage of each medication				
23. stated schedule for giving medications				
24. stated the need to keep the medication safe from the reach of her children				

FIG. 3 (continued)

SCREENING CRITERIA FOR TARGET POPULATION
RESPIRATORY DISTRESS:
Post-Discharge; Pneumonia and/or Bronchitis
1½ to 3 Years; No History of Chronic Illness/Anomalies
No Concurrent Illness

Page 1 of __1__

SCREENING CRITERIA	CLEARLY CHARTED MET	CLEARLY CHARTED NOT MET	INSUFFICIENT DATA FOR DECISION	SOURCE OF CRITERIA
ONE WEEK after discharge the PARENT				
1. stated symptoms of respiratory distress				
2. stated what to do if symptoms occur				
3. named each take-home medication				
4. stated side effects of each medication				
5. stated correct dosage for each medication				
6. stated schedule for giving medication				
7. stated the need to keep the medications safe from the reach of her children				
8. returned child to health care provider for follow-up care				
FOUR WEEKS after discharge the PATIENT				
9. interacted with parents in same level of attachment as preillness as validated by nurse with patient				

These model criteria are for screening patient care for subsequent peer review and do not constitute standards of care governing a nurse's or agency's obligation to a patient.

process, including audit and a comparison of results with the first audit, would be the action of choice.

REFERENCES

1. A. Donabedian, "Some Basic Issues in Evaluating the Quality of Health Care," in *Issues in Evaluative Research* (Kansas City, MO: American Nurses' Association, 1976), 3–28. Reprinted in L. T. Rinke, ed., *Outcome Measures in Home Care, Vol. I: Research* (New York: National League for Nursing, 1987), 3–28.

2. A more detailed description of a testing procedure is provided in the final report of the ANA-PSRO project, obtainable from the Bureau of Quality Assurance, 5600 Fishers Lane, Rockville, Maryland 20852.

Quality Assurance in Community Health Nursing

Beverly C. Flynn and Dixie W. Ray

Reprinted in full, this article by Flynn and Ray describes the state-of-the-art of outcome measures in the community/public health nursing practice field in the late 1970s.

Those of us in community health nursing, whether in faculty or service positions, are keenly aware of the need to document the effectiveness of community health nursing services. Pressures on agencies to provide such evidence come from a variety of sources such as third-party payers for Medicare and Medicaid, state and local community funding groups, state mandates and requirements, and legislators concerned with national health insurance and nursing's inclusion in PSROs. In essence, community health nursing is being forced to support its reason for being.

The question most frequently asked by funding sources and others is what methods of quality assurance are being used in community health nursing programs. To find answers, we surveyed the literature and contacted selected

Reprinted with permission from *Nursing Outlook,* 27 (October 1979), pp. 650–653, copyright © 1979, American Journal of Nursing Company.

This project was supported by USDHEW, Division of Nursing Special Project Grant Number 1 D10 NU 25042. This article was adapted from a speech given at the American Public Health Association Convention in Los Angeles, October, 1978.

agencies across the country, since we found that much of what is taking place in evaluating community health nursing services has not been published. In addition, we are involved in a six-state study, designed to find out what methods of quality assurance are being used in community health nursing programs in these states and to determine the feasibility of conducting research into quality assurance on a regional basis.

From the information we have obtained thus far from these community health nursing agencies, we will describe the methods being used in their patient care programs, discuss the benefits and issues relevant to quality assurance programs, and identify some directions for future efforts in quality assurance.

ONE REGION'S PROGRAMS

In Region V, which includes Illinois, Indiana, Michigan, Minnesota, Ohio, and Wisconsin, we found that the three most common methods used by official, home health, and combination agencies were record audits, supervisory review, and peer review. The record audits most frequently used were Phaneuf's, the National League for Nursing's (NLN) Home Health Agency Case Record Review, and locally developed ones.[1]

The Phaneuf method focuses on the legal definition of nursing practice and measures the process of care, utilizing discharge records. NLN's record review focuses on the adequacy of the nursing care plan and the appropriateness of the care provided. Other locally developed record audits measure outcomes or the results of care. Record audits in most agencies are usually conducted by peer review or intradisciplinary review committees. This finding is similar to that reported by Januska, Engel, and Wood in their survey of community health nursing programs in 1975.[2] The terms, supervisory and peer review, are confusing in that they are defined differently in agencies. For example, some agencies include observation as part of supervisory review and others do not, and some agencies include case conferences or the results of record audit as part of peer review.

An interesting difference, since the Januska et al. survey, is that agencies are increasing their efforts to develop outcome measures. For instance, the Minnesota Department of Health, Section of Community Nursing, has established a statewide data bank containing a total of 35 sets of core criteria and 128 individual sets of outcome criteria.[3] The Chicago VNA reported that it is developing scaled outcome criteria for 30 patient problems. Other agencies—the Cincinnati VNA and the Ramsey County Public Health Nursing Service in Saint Paul, Minnesota—report that they are measuring four outcome conditions. The Wisconsin Division of Health, Bureau of Community Health, has developed audit tools that are being tested with 12 to 15 agencies in conjunction with the problem-oriented record system.[4] These tools are unique in that they focus on both individual and family process and outcomes.

An interesting variation reported by four agencies is the involvement of consumers in evaluating community health nursing services. The Ramsey County Public Health Nursing Service has a consumer review committee, and three other agencies survey their consumers by questionnaire.

OTHER GEOGRAPHICAL AREAS

In four states outside of Region V—Pennsylvania, Delaware, Georgia, and South Carolina—problem-oriented records have been implemented as a first step in quality assurance. The Pennsylvania Assembly of Home Health Agencies focuses on patient outcomes through an examination of discharge records.[5] In this system, outcome audit criteria were developed for 12 audit topics, records were audited, variations from the criteria were identified, and decisions made about whether the variations were justified or were true deficiencies. Corrective action was then taken and reaudits were performed.

Progress in quality assurance in the other three states is at varying stages of development. In Delaware, after difficulties arose with the Phaneuf audit tool, four problems were identified and new audit tools were developed emphasizing outcomes. Both Georgia and South Carolina have developed standards for nursing care, utilizing ANA's *Guidelines for Nursing Care at the Local Level.*[6]

The Hartford VNA experienced difficulties similar to those in Delaware, finding problems with both the Phaneuf and NLN record audits. As a result, staff in this agency developed their own utilization review audit and are applying this tool for Medicare and Medicaid reimbursement. They have also developed a record process audit utilizing the ANA Guidelines noted above. It is their intent to develop outcome criteria and relate these to the process criteria.

The New Haven VNA has developed a patient classification system for its home care program, based on each patient's rehabilitation potential.[7] Patients are placed in one of five categories of care, each of which have predetermined and objectively measured outcomes. One of the benefits of this system is that each set of objectives and subobjectives for these categories is applicable to six disciplines providing home care.

The quality assurance program underway at the Omaha VNA has been presented at NLN and APHA meetings, and the creative work developed by this agency has had an impact on a number of community health nursing agencies. In this system, a taxonomy of 49 community health nursing problems were identified and are being tested in various sites in this country. The second phase of this VNA's project is to develop expected outcomes for these problems. Data are being gathered to identify what nurses think can be accomplished with clients having selected problems.

Another trend worth mentioning is computerized data collection or management information systems (MIS), as described by Saba and Levine.[8] For the most part, the emphasis in this system has been on statistical information and billing, not patient assessment and service evaluation. An exception is that home health agencies in South Carolina are computerizing clients' problems and those that are effectively handled by the community health nurse.

Additional quality assurance methods were reported by two agencies. The Tacoma Pierce County Health Department in Washington utilized self-evaluation and peer review, with observation of each community health nurse's practice and team participation as integral components of this process. The Hartford VNA conducts a patient satisfaction study that involves telephone interviews with patients to determine their perceptions of the care provided by various disciplines in the agency.

BENEFITS ACHIEVED

The agencies were able to identify a number of benefits as well as problems with, their quality assurance programs. For example, performance deficiencies among the various agency providers or staff have been identified, and inservice education has been designed and implemented to upgrade the level of skills of these workers. In the process of developing quality assurance programs, many agencies also needed to develop or update their policies, procedures, and protocols and communicate these changes to their staff.

At the same time, the new programs have provided information on staffing patterns that has been useful to staff and administration alike. Likewise, the programs have provided information needed to justify the expansion of services. In essence, the benefits of quality assurance programs not only have payoffs in terms of good management within agencies but also in terms of justifying community nursing services within the context of community resources. These are certainly steps in the right direction toward professional accountability.

RELEVANT ISSUES

On the other hand, there are many issues and difficulties with quality assurance programs in community health nursing today. Perhaps most important, programs are being developed and implemented in a very unsettled environment. On the state level, administrative reorganization has been going on over the last several years and, for the most part, nursing leadership in state health agencies has been seriously weakened. In addition, there has been a general lack of state administrative support for community health nursing services; this is manifested in austere spending, limiting the number of community health nurses and other employees. At the same time, some states have mandated that community health nurses must see increasing numbers of clients, as has been the case in South Carolina.

We have come to a point in our society where more isn't better and limits to growth must be set. However, federal and state legislation continues to be passed, requiring quality assurance endeavors such as the Early and Periodic Screening Diagnosis and Treatment Program (EPSDT), and Connecticut's mandatory quality assurance programs, with a target for implementing the process dimension by 1979, and outcome dimension by 1982. These factors create a snowball effect and result in a lack of coordination and fragmentation of quality assurance activities.

Other dilemmas result from a lack of distinction between quality of care and cost containment efforts. Porterfield claims that the PSRO legislation provides a mechanism to control costs under the guise of enhancing quality of care.[9]

Questions we need to address related to quality of care and cost containment include: What is the minimum level of quality we will accept? When do we say "no" to seeing more patients/families in order to maintain that level of quality? Will this create risks of losing funds? If patients/families don't achieve a certain level of outcome, will community health nursing services be reimbursed for the services given?

Compounding these issues is the fact that consumers and providers define quality of care differently, yet quality of care efforts are, for the most part, provider controlled. Consumers are the ones most concerned with quality health care as well as cost containment, but they have minimal, if any, input into the decisions about community health nursing services.

The definitions of terms in community health nursing and quality assurance are also most confusing. In attempting to clarify some of this confusion, Williams contrasted community health nursing to clinical nursing, which focuses on the individual or patient.[10] According to Williams, the community health nurse is concerned with the health status of many aggregates, the influence of environmental factors on the health of populations, and setting priorities for prevention and health maintenance strategies over curative ones. Seen from this perspective, community health nursing is clearly more than nursing individuals in the community.

Accompanying the confusion as to what constitutes community health nursing is the fact that there are deficiencies or lack of measurements for prevention and health promotion activities, as well as the impact of services on families, groups, and communities. Conflicts also arise with Medicare and Medicaid legislation, which requires documentation of the quality of care with the focus on the individual patient and the medical diagnosis or disease.

Another deficit we found is the limited number of community health nurses who have research expertise and who are involved in quality assurance programs. It is clear that neither the educational nor the practice arena has the resources needed to document the effectiveness of community health nursing practice. Service may lack research skills, personnel, money, and time, but academia lacks the reality of the work settings and practice experiences necessary to develop and validate criteria and data collection methods. While most of the quality assurance efforts are taking place in the larger agencies in this country, each is separately developing criteria and modifying methods for use in their programs. Rarely do they share experiences, and there is duplication of effort. Everyone is doing his own thing, explaining that the criteria and data collection methods are agency specific and not applicable in other areas. The smaller agencies are the most disadvantaged by this state of affairs; they are often geographically isolated and have the most limited resources.

As if these difficulties aren't enough, community health nurses themselves are creating another major problem. We found a fair amount of distrust and competition among community health nurses. These attitudes may be basic to human nature, but if we all share the goal of advancing quality assurance programs in community health nursing, we must decide: Do we want collaboration or competition within our ranks?

FUTURE DIRECTIONS

Perhaps our greatest priority is developing a partnership between community health nursing service and education, on the one hand, and the consumers of our services, on the other. With increasing financial and manpower constraints placed on agencies and educational institutions, community health nurses must conserve their scarce resources and work together to accomplish mutual goals. Quality assurance efforts prevent a unique opportunity for such collaborative efforts.

That is not to say it will be an easy task. On the contrary, sensitivity to the needs and concerns of the two sectors in community health nursing and their consumers must be openly addressed. An excellent example of collaborative efforts between service and education is the community survey done to assess the health needs of older adults by Managan and others.[11] Although this was not a quality assurance program, the results provide baseline data to examine the future impact of community health nursing services on a specific population within the context of the community.

Along this same line, quality assurance activities need to be coordinated within and across state boundaries. Such efforts would provide an environment in which quality assurance criteria and data collection methods could be developed, revised, and utilized on a regional basis. A trend in this direction is evident in the statewide efforts noted in South Carolina and Minnesota and with our feasibility study in Region V.

In developing these criteria, we should include such areas as levels of prevention, health status of many aggregates, the influence of environmental factors on the health of populations, community involvement in health, self-care or self-reliance, and active consumer participation. At the same time, improved methods of data collection are also needed. Questions are always raised about the reliability and validity of data-collecting instruments. Development and testing of these methods at the regional level will provide opportunities to establish reliability and validity that are unavailable to individual agencies. In addition to individual efforts, those of us in community health nursing should keep abreast of developments in related research areas. These include the health service field and the behavioral sciences, including psychology and sociology. We need to crtically examine the measures being used in these fields to determine their relevance to quality assurance in community health nursing.

Finally, community health nurses should make concerted efforts to work with groups formed to carry out legislative mandates such as those involved in developing and implementing criteria for quality assurance—for example, local, state, and national PSRO councils. These particular councils provide opportunities for non-physician provider membership and we should actively support nurses in filling these positions.

In summary, there are many directions in which community health nursing can collaboratively and individually work toward proving the worth of its services. We believe it is a challenge that those in education and service must resolve together.

ABOUT THE AUTHORS

At the time of writing, Beverly Flynn, PhD, RN, was professor and chairperson, and Dixie Ray, MPA, was lecturer, Department of Community Health Nursing, Indiana University, Indianapolis.

REFERENCES

1. M. C. Phaneuf, *The Nursing Audit: Profile for Excellence* (New York: Appleton-Century-Crofts, 1972); and *Utilization Review Guidelines for Home Health Agencies* (New York: National League for Nursing, Department of Public Health Nursing, 1971).

2. C. Januska, J. Engle, and J. Wood, "Status of Quality Assurance in Public Health Nursing" (Washington, DC: Public Health Nursing Section, American Public Health Association, 1976). Reprinted in L. Rinke, ed., *Outcome Measures in Home Care, Vol. I: Research* (New York: National League for Nursing, 1987), 55–77.

3. Frances Decker et al. "Using Patient Outcomes to Evaluate Community Health Nursing," *Nursing Outlook*, 27 (April 1979), 278–282.

4. Rosemary Vahldieck, "Nursing Audit in Community Health Agencies" (Madison: Bureau of Community Health, Wisconsin Division of Health, 1975) (mimeographed).

5. *Quality Assurance in Home Health Care* (Camp Hill, PA: Pennsylvania Assembly of Home Health Agencies, 1976).

6. *Guidelines for Review of Nursing Care at the Local Level* (Kansas City, MO: American Nurses' Association, 1976).

7. Elizabeth Daubert, "Patient Classification System and Outcome Criteria," *Nursing Outlook,* 27 (July 1979), 450–454.

8. V. K. Saba and E. Levine, "Management Information Systems for Public Health Community Health Agencies," paper presented at the Annual Meeting of the American Public Health Association, Miami Beach, Florida, October 18–21, 1976 (mimeographed).

9. J. D. Porterfield, "Evaluation of the Care of Patients: Codman Revisited," *Bulletin of the New York Academy of Medicine*, 52 (January 1976), 30–38.

10. C. A. Williams, "Community Health Nursing—What Is It?" *Nursing Outlook,* 25 (April 1977), 250–254.

11. Dorothy Managan et al. "Older Adults: A Community Survey of Health Needs," *Nursing Research,* 23 (September-October 1974), 426–432.

The 'Black Box'
of Home Care Quality

Charles P. Sabatino

In 1986, spurred by indictments of "sicker and quicker" discharges to the community because of the Medicare prospective payment system, the Administration on Aging of the U.S. Department of Health and Human Services supported an examination of the quality of in-home health services, conducted by the Commission on Legal Problems of the Elderly of the American Bar Association. Released under the title of The "Black Box" of Home Care Quality, *the American Bar Association's report assumes a critical, consumer-oriented approach to the issue of quality assurance in home care. Since this report has brought the public's attention to the issue of quality in home care services, it represents a significant policy perspective that must be taken into account. Excerpted here are the report's chapters addressing the definition of quality and delineating its recommendations.*

Excerpted with permission from *The "Black Box" of Home Care Quality,* a report presented by the Chairman of the Select Committee on Aging, U.S. House of Representatives, 99th Congress, Second Session, August 1986, prepared by the American Bar Association Commission on Legal Problems of the Elderly, Washington, DC. This project was supported, in part, by award number G-HHS 90AM0112/01, from the Administration on Aging, Office of Human Development Services, U.S. Department of Health and Human Services.

THE ELUSIVE CONCEPT OF QUALITY

What is Quality?

The concept of quality, even when economic considerations are put aside, is elusive. Quality has many dimensions which may vary with the viewpoint of the examiner.[1] Besides economic interpretations, there are physical, psychological, functional and social interpretations of quality. Most people will agree that high quality of care in basic terms means meeting the individual's medical, emotional, psychosocial, and rehabilitative needs and effectively encouraging his or her maximum functional independence. However, translating this ideal into operational standards is where the real difficulties begin.

A complete regulatory system contains not only appropriate quality standards but also two other components: a monitoring system and enforcement system. Even with all three components firmly in place, the system itself does not create quality. Ultimately, that can only come from the people and organizations that provide the care. The regulatory system at best provides only some crude measures of quality and a system of checks and balances to identify and stop clearly substandard or abusive services. Thus, regulation functions more as a negative prophylactic than as a positive insurance.

Compared to other components in the continuum of care, home care has an additional, unique problem with respect to regulation. Maintaining a person in his or her home does not just mean maintaining that person's health and functional ability in an objectively defined way; it also means maintaining his or her personal lifestyle to a far greater extent than is possible in any residential long-term care setting. Home care is the one health care setting where the provider comes into the patient/client's domain rather than vice versa.

The quality of *life* is really a dimension separate from quality of *care,* yet fundamental to a patient's well-being and to the whole philosophy of in-home care. Quality of life is also idiosyncratic to the patient/client in a way that conflicts with the notion of uniformity of standards and procedures.

It is noteworthy that the quality of life concept has also emerged as a key concern in the field of nursing home regulation reform. The Institute of Medicine, in its recent seminal report on improving the quality of care in nursing homes, recommends that quality of life, in addition to quality of care, be incorporated as a condition of participation in the Medicare program.[2]

To achieve quality of life objectives theoretically means finding criteria unique to each client. It is highly unlikely that a regulatory system could directly ensure this kind of process. Nevertheless, there may be ways that a regulatory system can orient itself sufficiently toward a goal of accountability to the individual client so as to make this process possible. This orientation toward client accountability will be discussed in more detail below.

Quality in Terms of Structure, Process, and Outcome

Theorists have generally recognized three basic traditional categories of quality of care standards in health care: structural, process, and outcome measures.[3] Structural standards focus upon the organization and framework for care, setting requirements for organizational form, facilities, and equipment, fiscal resources and management, number and qualifications of staff, and other such indices. Structural standards tend to measure an entity's capacity to deliver services rather than the quality of the actual services rendered.

Process standards focus on the actual procedures followed in delivering care and compare them to accepted norms for what good care should look like. Such standards for performance would, for example, require surveyors to examine a sample of cases to determine what happened during the care and treatment of that patient: Was an assessment done in accordance with prescribed requirements? Was an appropriate care plan devised and followed? Were the staff supervised as required? And so on.

Outcome measures are concerned with the end result of care: whether there is any measurable change (or stabilization) in the health or social status of the patient as a result of services rendered. Outcome measures are obviously easier to develop where there are discrete, changeable physical conditions being examined, as is common in hospitals or other acute care settings. Outcome measurements for chronic conditions and mental or physical functional limitations are harder to come by, although still conceptually feasible.

Each of these three categories of standards possess inherent strengths and weaknesss which make them helpful but by no means complete measures of quality. Structural measures have been the primary component of the Medicare Conditions of Participation for home health agencies and more so for skilled nursing facilities. Advocates for nursing home residents have even challenged the nursing home survey process, in part, for this reason, pointing out that of some 541 items on the federal inspection form fewer then 30 were even marginally related to patient care or required any patient observation.[4] It is not difficult to see why structural mechanisms have been so favored in the regulatory process—they can be surveyed primarily by a review of paper and perhaps an interview with an administrator. This is the easiest kind of function for a monitoring agency to perform. And, it has been justified on the assumption that if the provider of care has the capacity to provide good care, in all likelihood it will provide good care. Unfortunately, the assumption is not always borne out by experience.

Process standards have the advantage of examining actual care given, yet they are still limited in fundamental ways. Since every procedure and activity is expected to be documented in some way, this form of quality assessment also tends to rely heavily on paper review. Moreover, performance measures need to define the technically correct steps and decisions a provider must make. In long-term care, as contrasted to acute care, process standards are difficult to validate. The client's medical problems are typically chronic and multiple, and the client's social/personal/lifestyle needs (i.e., quality of life) are of greater importance than in acute care settings.

Outcome measures may be the most rationally sound form of measure; but the further one moves from examining purely medical outcomes, the more difficult it is to develop valid measures of outcome. Even where validated outcomes are measureable, the failure to achieve the desired outcome is not enough on which to base any conclusion about quality. One would still need to look at the whole process of care to see whether there were any legitimate reasons why the outcome was not achieved. Outcome-oriented quality assurance audits have been attempted by both the Colorado and Florida Association of Home Health Agencies and by the Public Health Nursing Section of the Minnesota Department of Health. They follow a traditional medical model by organizing patient care review around specific medical diagnoses with the assessment based on a comprehensive range of identifiable outcomes.

Both process and outcome standards have the additional problem of being time consuming, and therefore, expensive to develop, and even more so to carry out. Regulating bodies may have neither the requisite skills, manpower, or funds to carry out effective surveying and monitoring schemes. All three approaches primarily depend for their implementation upon the functioning of some kind of well-trained, third-party watchdog. The watchdog may be a state health department, the state licensing agency, an accrediting body, professional review organization, or the federal government itself.

Focusing on Accountability to the Consumer

The home care consumer, who is by definition physically or mentally dependent to some degree, is heavily dependent upon the regulatory system at all stages of the regulatory process: at the standard-setting stage (deciding what good care is), at the monitoring stage (evaluating the care given), and at the enforcement stage (taking corrective action when care is poor). While this dependency is inherent in the consumer protection underpinnings of the regulatory system, it also points out the lack of attention given to ways to directly empower the consumer within the regulatory framework. The traditional regulatory response has been to empower, sometimes quite unsuccessfully, a regulating agency. The care provider becomes accountable to some form of bureaucracy and not necessarily to the consumer.

Accountability to the consumer plays a potentially central role in any model of checks and balances for quality assurance in home care. It should be a fundamental value and goal in home care regulation, not because it is a substitute for structural, process or outcome mechanisms, but because it has been a largely deemphasized strategy and neglected value. It is a goal that acknowledges that quality in home care is uniquely client-specific and therefore should be controlled by the patient/client to the maximum extent feasible. To the extent that the goal of accountability to the consumer can be translated into a regulatory scheme, it holds the potential of increasing quality monitoring and enforcement without necessarily increasing regulatory bureaucracy.

RECOMMENDATIONS

1. Wider Applicability of Standards

Existing standards for licensure, certification, accreditation and other forms of quality assurance apply to differing slices of the home care field. A large portion of home care services need meet no standards whatsoever. A fundamental policy goal should be to establish as nearly universal a system of standards and quality control as possible—one that cuts across agency types and funding sources. On the state level, an option would be to establish or extend a licensure system to all home care services intended to maintain sick or functionally impaired persons in their homes. Presently, most state licensure is limited to traditionally medically oriented home health agencies. On the federal level, an option would be to strengthen what are now called the Medicare Conditions of Participation and to expand their applicability to any home care service or agency receiving federal funds. This would, at a minimum, encompass programs funded wholly or in part by Medicare, Medicaid, Social Services Block Grants, and the Older Americans Act.

2. Strengthening the Content of Standards

Current examples of home care standards focus heavily on agency structure, policy, and procedure—characteristics which pertain more to the capacity of the agency to provide good care than to the actual care given. Compliance often depends more on completing paperwork correctly than on performing the actual care with quality.

Improved and strengthened standards are needed, which not only measure basic structural and procedural characteristics but also focus on patient-worker interactions and quantifiable outcomes of care.

3. Bonding and Insurance

In order to provide a baseline of protection for consumers for loss or injury caused by negligence or misconduct of a home care worker, home care regulations should mandate minimum bonding and liability insurance requirements.

4. Consumer Empowerment

The home care regulatory system should recognize accountability to the consumer as a fundamental goal. Consumer empowerment strategies require an examination of at least five elements:

Patient/Client Rights. These should articulate in some detail basic individual rights and liberties (e.g., rights to courtesy and respect, privacy, confidentiality, security, freedom from abuse, non-discrimination) and specific care protocols (e.g., involvement in creating and evaluating a written care plan, the right to refuse treatment or services, the right to have properly trained staff, and coordination of all services).

Disclosure Requirements. Disclosure protocols are aimed essentially at educating patient/clients so that they have the information and knowledge they need to make decisions and act in their best interest. Disclosure protocols include matters such as a description of agency services; information about alternative services avilable in the community; costs and billing statements, regardless of source of payment; worker's and supervisor's name and number; advance notice of changes in services; patient/client rights; and grievance procedures.

Grievance Mechanisms. Effective grievance mechanisms are essential and should be formulated with the characteristics of the consumer foremost in mind. Sickness, impaired ability, and significant dependency on one's caretakers all create enormous disincentives against voicing criticism or pursuing complaints. To remedy this imbalance, supports and incentives should be built into the system to facilitate and, in some respects, encourage its use by clients. Procedures need to be easily understandable and simple to trigger.

One possible strategy would be to require regular surveys of clients to elicit comments and complaints. This function could be performed by a supervisor, or more preferably, by a nonemployee of the agency, such as an outside case manager or client advocate.

To enable clients to pursue remedies once problems are uncovered, policymakers should consider building into the system a patient/client advocacy resource that has the standing and authority to seek remedies and sanctions. A state ombudsman program or publicly funded patient advocate could provide the vehicle for such a function.

Finally, grievances and their documented outcomes need to be tied directly into the monitoring/evaluation function of the regulatory system, so that they become one of the determinants of the agency's licensure or certification status.

Consumer Input in Program Evaluation. The Medicare regulations and most state licensure schemes require some form of annual program evaluation to be performed by home care agencies. Medicare and several states require some consumer involvement in the process but do not define that involvement in any way. Consumer input in the evaluation process should be expressly incorporated into program evaluation in two ways. First, consumer involvement on the evaluating team should be specifically defined in terms of selection, authority, and number or proportion. Second, the data collected for review should include a defined representative sampling of clients who are solicited for their assessment of the care received. Both active and closed cases should be included, and family members should be surveyed where the patient/client is unavailable or unable to respond.

Consumer Policy Voice. Advisory bodies to individual agencies and to regulating entities should include defined levels of consumer participation. These bodies provide direction and advice on matters of standard setting, policy, program operation and monitoring. To foster consumer participation, more than just an invitation is necessary, for participation may be impeded by physical handicaps or lack of resources. Therefore, the system may need to provide for transportation, interpreters, personal care attendants, or other resources necessary to enable consumers to participate in advisory group functions.

5. Monitoring

The quality assurance monitoring function of the regulatory system should have both a periodic component (usually annual inspections) and a responsive component (triggered by a complaint or other evidence of quality problems). The monitoring process itself should expand its focus beyond the traditional structure, policy, and document review to include client-centered review, wherein monitors directly survey both clients and workers. An instructive model for this may be found in the Institute of Medicine's recommendations for improving quality of care in nursing homes.[5]

Since one of the recommendations of this report is the establishment of a quality assurance system that cuts across all agency types and funding sources, a new form of monitoring entity should be considered. A possible model is the use of an interdisciplinary, independent entity, having the necessary expertise available to evaluate both the professional and nonprofessional, medical and nonmedical services included under home care.

With respect to its responsive component, the monitoring system should be complemented by an ombudsman type consumer-oriented entity. This may be accomplished by expanding the jurisdiction and resources of existing nursing home ombudsman programs to include home care, or creating a patient advocate program specific to home care.

6. Sanctions

The range of formal sanctions available to enforce quality of care problems is most commonly limited to denial, revocation, or suspension of an agency's status, whether it be licensure, certification or accreditation. A strong system of accountability requires a flexible range of administrative and judicial enforcement sanctions. Additional administrative sanctions should include the ability to impose restricted or provisional licenses, pending correction of deficiencies and civil fines. Fines should be commensurate to the seriousness of violations and costly enough to encourage compliance. Judicial sanctions include injunctive relief to require compliance and criminal sanctions for serious violations. An additional option is a receivership sanction, under which a court may temporarily appoint a "receiver" to assume management of an agency in serious trouble in cases where continuation of client care is essential.

While not a sanction in a formal sense, the public disclosure and dissemination of information about agencies out of compliance with required standards is recommended as a way of enhancing the impact of the formal sanction. It is a tool aimed at increasing consumers' market power through information about provider quality.

Finally, the system of sanctions should grant recipients of home care a "private right of action" enabling consumers and advocates for consumers or groups representing consumers to sue providers that do not meet minimum required standards.

7. Education and Training

Homemaker-home health aides, personal care attendants and other non-professional or paraprofessional workers who provide the bulk of day-to-day supportive services in the home are largely untrained or undertrained. At a minimum, homemaker-home health aides and personal care attendants (or functionally similar personnel) should be required to complete an established and approved course of instruction, provided through a recognized educational entity such as a community college, leading to certification or licensure of the individual. Minimum orientation and in-service training requirements for all personnel should also be mandated.

8. Research and Data Collection

Our present state of knowledge about the home care field and about quality of home care services is inadequate. Research and improved data collection on all aspects of home care are needed, especially with respect to improving the accountability of services to the consumer and public. Public regulation of home care must contain adequate flexibility and incentives to encourage research and experimentation in new forms of services and their delivery, the monitoring of these services, and, in all cases, the evaluation of the quality of these services.

ABOUT THE AUTHOR

Charles P. Sabatino, JD, is Associate Staff Director, American Bar Association Commission on Legal Problems of the Elderly, Washington, DC.

REFERENCES

1. A. Donabedian, "Evaluating the Quality of Medical Care," *Milbank Memorial Fund Quarterly,* 44 (1966), 166–206.
2. Institute of Medicine, *Improving the Quality of Care in Nursing Homes* (Washington, DC: National Academy Press, 1986).
3. E. Layzer, "Regulation of Homemaker-Home Health Aide Services" (Waltham, MA: Levinson Policy Institute, Brandeis University, December 1977), 52–58; and Donabedian, "Evaluating the Quality of Medical Care," 168–170.
4. Smith v. Heckler, 747 F.2d 583, 588 (10th Cir. 1984), *rev'g* Smith v. O'Halloran, 557 F.Supp 289 (D. Colo. 1983).
5. Institute of Medicine, *Improving the Quality of Care in Nursing Homes.*

Part 2

Promulgated Standards

Model Standards: A Guide for Community Preventive Health Services

In 1986, the American Public Health Association, in collaboration with several other organizations, published a second edition of its Model Standards. *Like the ANA* Guidelines for Review of Nursing Care at the Local Level, *published a decade earlier, the APHA publication provides a framework for developing service standards. Excerpted here are sections of the APHA document that describe the theoretical and practical background to the standards offered. Although most of the areas included in the APHA document address preventive health services, the publication includes a section on home health services, which is reprinted here.*

HOW TO USE THE MODEL STANDARDS

Flexibility

The principal feature of the community preventive health services standards is flexibility.

It is clear that significant differences do occur among the thousands of communities of the United States in the mix of preventive diseases and health conditions facing those communities, the range of preventive health services

Excerpted with permission of the American Public Health Association from *Model Standards: A Guide for Community Preventive Health Services,* 2nd ed., a collaborative project of the American Public Health Association, Association of State and Territorial Health Officials, National Association of County Health Officials, United States Conference of Local Health Officers, and U.S. Department of Health and Human Services, Public Health Service, Centers for Disease Control, copyright © 1985, American Public Health Association, Washington, DC.

available to them, and the financial resources available to each community to provide such services. This disparity of services and resources is unfortunate, but is, nevertheless, fact.

Because of the existence of these significant variations, the standards in this document have been designed to permit quantification of objectives at the community level so that negotiated, incremental achievement can be predicted and realized for each individual community. In addition, the standards have been developed with the necessary flexibility to assist in program area priority setting and to accommodate budgetary realities. Some objectives allow for less flexibility than others, recognizing that certain objectives are so basic for protection of the public's health that significant variances are hard to defend. While one of the obvious uses of these standards is the generation of objective programmatic data which can be presented as budget justification, it is also true that without significant new resources, these same data can assist in assignment of priorities to assure greater yield from existing programs.

The Negotiation Process

The most striking feature which will be noted in the standards that follow is the recurring use of a series of blank spaces. These blank spaces have been provided throughout this document for such diverse factors as dates, disease entities, institutional settings, environmental agents, vaccines or other immunizing agents, and quantifiable measures. This system provides the necessary flexibility to accommodate existing local conditions while stimulating incremental improvement in even the best of community service settings. "Filling in blanks" is the work of the contemplated negotiation process for each program area. Through assessment of community need and identification of available resources, the program area priorities will be developed and incremental improvement objectives will be established.

No less frequently than once every other year, state officials with specific program responsibility should meet with their local counterparts to review existing programs, program needs, potential resources, and existing agreements. Following that review, both parties will need to agree upon the specific material to be inserted in each black space for the upcoming program year or for each of two subsequent program years.

Once the negotiating parties have reached such agreement, the results of their deliberations should be made available for public review and comment. While the official health agency will most frequently be the lead agency in each of the program areas addressed by these standards, the Preamble indicates the importance of input from other governmental agencies, the private and voluntary sectors, and other interested individuals and community organizations in the ultimate quantification of program objectives. After receipt, review, and consideration of all such comment, the program negotiating parties will need to make appropriate amendments to their original proposals and finalize their agreements for the following year(s).

In agreeing upon specific quantifiable measures for each community, a continuing interaction is anticipated among local, state, and federal agencies. For example, a national outcome objective may have been established for a specific program area. If that is the case, prior negotiations between state and federal officials may have established the contribution of each state toward meeting that national goal. The state, in turn, in its negotiations with its communities, will need to assure that the combined efforts of all community programs in the state meet or exceed its agreed-to contribution to the national effort.

In other program areas where national outcome measures have not been proposed, the negotiation process will be between appropriate state and local program officials—always with an eye toward improving the health status of the community.

In a few program areas, the state is the direct provider of local services. In such instances, the state should review its own program accomplishments and propose specific outcomes for the next program year. These proposals, as well as those negotiated between state and local program officials, should be made available for public review and comment, and appropriate modification made as necessary.

Finally, in a few program areas (most notably air quality, safe drinking water, and wastewater management), federal statute or regulation has already set the dates for achievement of specific outcome measures. Such conditions must, of course, be recognized in any negotiation process.

Modifications for Local Need

Throughout the document, efforts have been made to assure completeness. However, the document should in no way be considered as exhaustive or exclusionary. As discussed in the Preamble, even the program areas selected for inclusion cannot be considered as an exhaustive catalog of community need for preventive health services. Obviously, additional program areas may be considered as state or local needs and programming dictate.

The same caveat applies to outcome and process objectives delineated for each program. State and local needs may dictate expansion in any given program.

It is in the realm of "indicators," however, that there exists the greatest need for modification to meet unique state and local conditions. For example, the single word "existence" is frequently employed as an indicator for a specific objective. Clearly, this is an imcomplete and insufficient indicator without further definition. Such definition is an appropriate corollary to the negotiation process described above. Factors such as quantification, quality control and evaluation will need to be considered and agreed to by the negotiating parties whenever an indicator appears which lacks such precision. In addition, all indicators may not apply in their stated format to a given community without further refinement. For example, a stated indicator may be more appropriate on an age, race, sex-adjusted, or specific basis. This, too, should be considered at the time of program negotiation.

Finally, the terms "incidence" and "prevalence" have been employed as indicators. Recognizing that these terms depend on both accuracy of diagnosis or interpretation and completeness of reporting, they are used, nonetheless, as reasonable barometers of community health status. Significant changes in any variable contributing to the determination of "incidence" or "prevalence" in a community should be or should become readily apparent to the program area negotiating parties, and taken into account in their future negotiations.

Data Needs

The objectives of the standards for many program areas address preventive health services available throughout both the private and public sectors. Data on their attainment should therefore apply to the total defined population in need, regardless of the source of the service.

In fact, however, current data systems are often unable to provide these data or documentation for the private sector and, in some cases, the public sector as well. It is feasible to expect local agencies to identify these data needs and to project future sources of data for program areas in which they are involved. However, at this time, some standards may be measurable only for the public sector component. Thus, developing a community-oriented surveillance and epidemiology system capable of acquiring the necessary data from both the public and private sectors is the key to successful application of the standards. A specific epidemiology and surveillance standard, therefore, is included in the package of standards.

Cross References

Throughout the standards document, cross-references are made from one program area to another. This process indicates the clear interrelation between and among program areas.

One critically important cross-reference appears with each standard relating that standard to the section on Administration and Supporting Services. The standard for Administration and Supporting Services, unlike the others in the document, was developed principally for the official community health agency.

Certain elements of this standard, however (e.g., manpower, fiscal management, program planning and evaluation), have direct application to each of the other program areas, and should be considered as appropriate objectives for each standard.

While cross-referencing has been included in an attempt to be of assistance to users of the document, the cross-referencing should not be considered to be exhaustive.

MODEL STANDARDS
AREA: HOME HEALTH SERVICES

Goal: A full range of preventive, therapeutic, and long-term home health services will be delivered within the community so that appropriate home care services are available and utilized as a responsible, feasible and desired alternative to institutionalization. Residents of the community with illnesses or handicaps which restrict self-care but do not require acute care or continuous supervision will be able to continue living at home rather than in a health care institution for as long as desirable and feasible.

Focus	Objectives	Indicators
	Outcome	
	O-1 By 19__, __ percent of persons known to be in need of non-institutional supportive services will receive the appropriate level of services.	Percent of persons in need of services who receive them.
	O-2 By 19__ the percent of inappropriate placements in long-term care institutions will not exceed __.	Percent of inappropriate placements.
	Process	
Long-Term Care	**P-1** By 19__, __ percent of persons medically qualified for institutional placement will actually be cared for in the appropriate home care setting.	a. Hospital, long-term care, mental health, and home health agency records relative to admission, discharge and community placement. b. Presence of adequate hospital long-term care discharge planning program.

Focus	Objectives	Indicators
	1a By 19__, __ percent of persons being considered for long-term institutional placement will receive an assessment of health, social, financial and other factors to determine the acceptability and feasibility of receiving needed care in the home. Such assessments will be done prior to admission to the institution.	
	1b By 19__, __ percent of persons admitted to nursing homes will have had pre-admission assessments documenting that they are appropriately placed and could not have been adequately cared for in the home.	
	1c 19__, __ percent of persons in long-term care and mental health institutions will be periodically considered for community placement.	
	P-2 By 19__ the mental hospital readmission rate of selected mental health clients will be reduced to __ percent through provision of assessment, counseling and in home services in support of mental health outpatient services.	Mental health facility readmission rates.
	Cross Reference: Aging and Dependent Populations, Institutional Services, Mental Health	

Focus	Objectives	Indicators
Hospice	**P-3** By 19__, __ percent of persons and families in need of hospice care will receive that care from a home-hospice program structured to minimize institutionalization.	Hospital, hospice, and home health agency records.
Acute Care	**P-4** By 19__, __ percent of persons convalescing from specified surgical procedures, medical events, and/or medical interventions will convalesce in the home with needed patient monitoring, dressing changes, and other necessary services provided in the home. *Cross Reference:* Institutional Services	Hospital and home health agency records.
	P-5 By 19__, __ percent of antenatal and postnatal patients at high risk of complication potentially preventable by in-home counseling, health education, or home-health services will receive such services. *Cross Reference:* Maternal and Child Health	Physician and hospital referrals.
Preventive Services for Adults	**P-6** By 19__, __ percent of persons experiencing repeated hospital admissions for a chronic health condition will receive a home health assessment and neces-	Hospital records.

Focus	Objectives	Indicators
	sary home health services to minimize both the frequency of readmission and length of each admission. *Cross Reference:* Chronic Disease Control, Institutional Services	
Availability and Accessibility of Services	**P-7** By 19__ home care services necessary to meet client and family needs will be available and accessible to all those in need.	a. Volume of service and profile of clients served compared to demographic profile of community. b. Presence of mechanisms to assure availability and access to those unable to pay.
	7a By 19__ nursing and selected other home health services will be available, at least on an emergency basis, 24 hours a day, seven days a week, including holidays.	Presence of coverage.
*	**7b** By 19__ the community will have access to ____ home health services. *Insert specific home health service, e.g., a. Nursing b. Home health aide c. Homemaker d. Personal care aide e. Physical, occupational, speech, and hearing therapy f. Hyperalimentation g. Intravenous fluids h. Social work i. Financial assessment	Presence of services.

Focus	Objectives	Indicators
	j. Nutrition counseling k. Home delivered meals l. Transportation m. Respite care n. Medical equipment o. Home renovation p. In-home comprehensive client assessment q. Case management r. MCH preventive services s. Preventive services for adults t. Hospice services u. Environmental health services (in-home safety, and sanitation assessment)	
Community and Professional Awareness	**P-8** By 19__ the community will be served by a program to increase community and professional awareness of the availability, range, and sources of home health services and their appropriate utilization.	a. Existence of information and referral program in community. b. Number of referrals from acute long-term care and mental health facilities to home health agencies. c. Number of referrals to agency from noninstitutional sources: family, self, community agencies.
Quality Assurance	**P-9** By 19__ programming to assure the quality of home health services will be in place.	a. Agency licensure and/or certification. b. Staff certification. c. Utilization review committee. d. Other quality assurance studies as appropriate.

Standards of
Home Health Nursing Practice

In accordance with its goal of providing professional practice standards addressing the wide variety of clinical nursing practice fields, the American Nurses' Association published Standards of Home Health Nursing Practice *in 1986. Originally, ANA standards were developed around the nursing process framework. As seen in this excerpt addressing the nursing process component of intervention, ANA has broadened its approach to the development of standards to address structure, process, and outcome criteria.*

STANDARD VI: INTERVENTION

The nurse, guided by the care plan, intervenes to provide comfort, to restore, improve, and promote health, to prevent complications and sequelae of illness, and to effect rehabilitation.

Rationale

The nurse implements the care plan to achieve the desired goals and objectives. The nurse provides direct care, incorporates preventive measures in the client's care, teaches the family and nonprofessional caregivers methods to promote the client's recovery, and provides comfort and support during a terminal illness.

Structure Criteria

1. The nurse is the case manager.

2. A mechanism exists to provide the intial and periodic assessment of client needs by a registered nurse to assure safe, adequate, and appropriate care.

3. Independent nursing functions are employed to enhance the medical treatment plan and enrich the services provided to the client.

4. A mechanism exists for reviewing staffing patterns and revising them in accord with client care needs.

5. Intervention skills are maintained and increased through professional development.

Process Criteria

The nurse generalist—

1. Implements interventions that are based on applicable scientific theories.

2. Intervenes with the concurrence and/or participation of the client and family.

3. Administers medically prescribed medications and treatments.

4. Treats physical and psychological responses to changes in health status, level of independence, and treatments.

5. Teaches prevention or control of disease progression or disability.

6. Coordinates client services provided by other health professionals while serving as an advocate for the client and family.

7. Supervises and evaluates ancillary personnel who provide care to clients and families.

8. Informs the client and family about the client's health status, health care resources, and treatments.

9. Teaches the client and family self-care concepts and skills.

10. Reviews interventions and revises them in accord with responses of the client and family.

11. Ensures continuity of care.

12. Documents interventions and responses of the client and family.

In addition, the nurse specialist functions as a consultant to the nurse generalist in nursing interventions.

Outcome Criteria

1. The client and family demonstrate self-care to the extent of their ability.
2. There is measurable evidence of progress toward goal achievement.
3. The client and family use community resources appropriately.
4. Problems, interventions, and responses of the client and family are recorded in a systematic, retrievable, and timely manner.
5. There is documented evidence that interdisciplinary services are in accord with client needs and capability.

Position Statement:
Productivity Expectations

Michigan Home Health Assembly

As a final example of promulgated standards developed by an organization, included here is a position statement issued by the Michigan Home Health Assembly. This statement of practice standards reflects the synthesis of ideal professional practice standards with the constraints imposed by actual service delivery in the field. Note that the outcome statements address parameters of knowledge, skill, and health status that are common threads in service and agency outcome standards.

The home health care industry is concerned with increasing costs in provision of services coupled with limitations in reimbursement. Individual agencies are exploring options to control costs and increase staff productivity. The Michigan Home Health Assembly, representing the home health industry in Michigan, requested that its Clinical Services Committee explore the impact of increased productivity requirements on the quality of home care services.

The Clinical Services Committee encourages those agencies planning to implement minimal requirements and monitor staff productivity to consider the following factors:

Reprinted with permission of the Michigan Home Health Assembly, Lansing, MI.

1. An overall high acuity level of patient illness that has occurred in part from early discharge from the acute care setting.

2. Excessive paperwork requirement necessitated by governmental regulations and third-party payer.

3. Time requirements for coordination of services with multiple health care providers related to complex patient problems.

4. Lack of patient/family education or retention of learning prior to admission to home health care.

5. Advanced level of knowledge and skills required by the home health nurse necessitated by treatments using high technology and specialized equipment.

6. Time required to travel to patient's place of residence that is influenced by urban or rural setting to the area of agency services.

These factors should impact significantly on the visit standard set by the agency. As agencies explore quantitative expectations, quality should not be overlooked. Although quality is difficult to define, certain outcomes indicate whether quality services have been provided. These outcomes include:

1. The patient/family is knowledgeable of and participates in their health care plan of treatment.

2. There is an improvement in the ability of the patient/caregiver to perform the patient's activities of daily living (e.g., mobility, personal hygiene, nutritional intake, etc.).

3. Plan for alternatives has been established for care if #2 is not met.

4. Patient and family have received information and/or have been referred to available community resources.

5. A potential exists for a reduction in the episodic use of high-cost health care (e.g., hospitalization, emergency room use, etc.).

Agencies have a responsibility to develop home visit expectations within a time-frame for attainment of specified outcomes. Each home health agency must determine their individual productivity expectations based on the variable identifed in order to provide quality patient care.

Part 3

Programmatic Approaches

A Model for Evaluating
a Community Health Agency

Mabel H. Morris

Integration of planning, implementation, and overall evaluation is a challenge for most community health agencies. Updated specially for this volume, this article provides an excellent model for agency evaluation, emphasizing the achievement and maintenance of consistent interrelationships in a community health agency as a total operational system. The article provides a conceptual model that may be applied to planning, implementing, and evaluating a system of health care services. It focuses on overall health and cost outcomes in relation to structure, process, and intermediate outcomes. Morris describes how to focus agency administration and internal operations in a cohesive feedback system, making certain that measurable agency objectives and activities that support the objectives function together to meet the health care needs of the community served.

Today, the consumers and purchasers of health care services want to know whether they are getting quality care for their health care dollars, how much it costs, and what good it is doing. This paper will describe an evaluation

This is a revised version of a paper published in *Community Health—Today and Tomorrow,* copyright © 1979, National League for Nursing, New York, pp. 15-36.

method that can assist administrators and their staffs to develop credible answers to these questions.

BACKGROUND INFORMATION

In 1972, Community Nursing Services (CNS) of Philadelphia was awarded a contract by the Division of Nursing, Health Resources Administration, U.S. Department of Health, Education, and Welfare. The purpose of the contract was to develop and test a computerized record system that would identify, analyze, store and summarize information relevant to administrative decision making, planning, and evaluation of public health nursing services.

In its initial efforts to fulfill the purpose and requirements of the contract, the project staff of CNS engaged in an extensive search of the literature as well as discussions with consumers, community health care administrators, agency staff at all levels of decision making, and national, regional, state, and local authorities in health and health-related fields. The purpose of these activities was to identify what information was relevant to administrative decision making, planning, and evaluation of public health nursing services.

As a result of this exploration, the project staff identified three types of information considered by the majority of persons consulted as relevant to administrators of any health care system:

1. Information that can provide concrete evidence of an agency's ability to deliver accessible, quality health care as planned and to achieve predefined health and cost outcomes in target populations.

2. Information that can serve as the basis for improving administrative planning, evaluation, decision making, and action in operational health care settings.

3. Information that can meet an agency's internal and external reporting requirements.

In its search of the literature, members of the project staff found a number of successful methods for acquiring the third type of information but less on the second type and no published evidence of a successful attempt to acquire the first type. The staff also found that consumers and payers of health care services were exerting considerable pressure on health care agencies for the first type. The project director and project officer both agreed that all three types of information were necessary to meet the public's demand for information and the agency's need to be accountable. However, the project staff had to concentrate most of its efforts on the first type of information.

According to authorities on program evaluation, acquiring information on whether and how an agency is delivering accessible, quality health care services and achieving desired health and cost outcomes in target populations requires administrators to, first, establish a system that is capable of doing what is intended and second, build in a method for generating data that will provide continuous evidence of how well the system is performing compared to what was planned.

Authorities also agree that establishing such a system requires the identification of the parameters to be studied, the establishment of desired relationships between and among the parameters, the definition of accessible, quality health care and desired health and cost outcomes in operational terms, and the selection of criteria against which to measure performance and accomplishments.[1]

In the past, it has been considered difficult to meet all these requirements because of the numerous, complex variables involved and the lack of universal agreement on the definition of terms and the measures of performance and accomplishments. Given the present advances in systems theory and computer technology, the difficulty in organizing and managing numerous variables is no longer a major problem. Disagreement on the definition of terms and measures of performance and accomplishments need not be an issue as long as there is internal consistency. In fact, the differences in community needs and agency purposes may require some agencies to define terms differently.

The major difficulty for members of the project staff in their efforts to establish a system capable of delivering accessible, quality health care was the lack of a conceptual framework for guiding a complex thought process. This difficulty seemed to be due to the complexity of a total and dynamic health care system in which there are many uncontrollable variables that are not conducive to traditional evaluation designs.

In the last year of the contract, the staff discovered a system control model for evaluating health programs that provided a framework for moving systematically through complex processes using the best scientific knowledge and methods available to establish new health care systems or assess and revise existing systems. Because of time constraints, the project staff was only able to demonstrate the feasibility of using the model and its components to establish a system capable of doing what was planned. However, the population was small—185 patients or families. In addition, all of the criteria and standards were not tested for reliability. Consensus among recognized authorities on the appropriateness of the theory underlying the operational plan was not obtained, and training manuals were not developed.

In spite of these limitations, the project staff was very excited about the practical and realistic nature of the model for use in an operational setting. After the project was terminated, the Project Director, Mrs. Margaret Kauffman, the Project Officer, Dr. O. Marie Henry, and the author as the Regional Nurse Consultant continued to refine and clarify the use of the model for improving administrative planning, evaluation, and decision making in a larger population.

In 1982, a new proposal was submitted to complete the unfinished activities in a larger population. This proposal was approved but unfunded by the federal government due to budget constraints. Although we continued to collaborate on refining the model, changes in our work assignments reduced the continuity of our efforts.

The following description of the model and its use represents the most recent status of efforts to operationalize the model. For purposes of this paper the description will be that of a community health nursing agency. However, we believe that the process can be used in any health care delivery system.

THE BASIC MODEL AND A MODIFIED VERSION

Figure 1 illustrates the basic system control model as described by Dr. Rita Zemach, then Associate Professor, Department of Biotatistics, University of Michigan.[2] According to Zemach, this model is based on system dynamics and control theory.

A *system* is defined as a set of parts designed and coordinated to achieve a set of objectives. *System dynamics* is concerned, first, with establishing a social unit capable of achieving objectives rather than simply with the achievement of objectives themselves. *Control theory,* on the other hand, is concerned with finding some rational way to assure that what an agency considers to be the most desirable mode of operation for achieving its objectives is indeed being carried out as planned.

Although Figure 2 represents a modified version of the basic model, these two concepts—system dynamics and control theory—have been retained. The modifications include some changes in the terminology describing the components of the basic model in order to conform to terms more familiar to community health care workers and thereby facilitate communications. In addition, a mechanism was added for the continuous feedback of information on the appropriateness of an agency's internal operations. This was done to ensure that the services are being delivered as planned or that timely corrective action can be taken.

The terms *overall health* and *cost outcomes* were substituted for the term *output.* This was done to ensure that health status and cost outcomes will be the focus of evaluation rather than process activities or outputs. Finally, questions were added to the modified version of the model as a guide for achieving and maintaining consistent interrelationships among all components of the model during the planning process.

The parts or components of the model as modified and shown in Figure 2 are as follows:

FIGURE 1
Control System Employing Feedback and Feedforward of Information

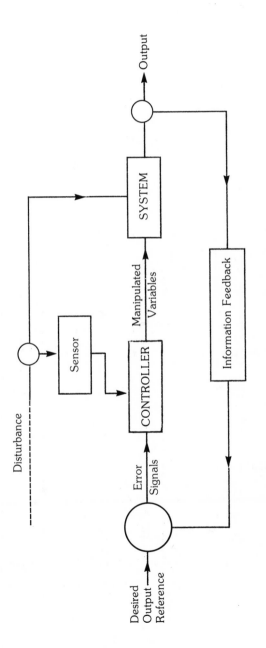

Source: Rita Zemach, "Program Evaluation and System Control," *American Journal of Public Health*, 63 (July 1973), 608.

FIGURE 2
Illustration of a Modified System Control Model for Evaluation of a Community Health Care Agency

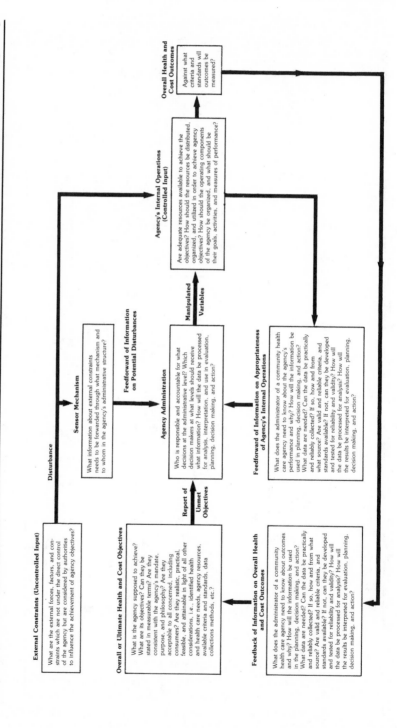

1. *The overall or ultimate health and cost objectives,* or operational, measurable statements of what an agency expects to accomplish in the health status of the target population and the cost of doing so. These objectives should be based on identified needs of the target population. They should also be interrelated consistently with other agency statements of philosophy, purpose and policies.

2. *External constraints (uncontrolled inputs),* or those personal and environmental factors that are inputs not under an agency's direct control but which, under certain circumstances, can contribute to or interfere with health or the delivery of health care and thereby affect an agency's performance and the achievement of desired objectives. These factors include such personal characteristics of a population as age, sex, race, residence, socioeconomic status, culture, health and medical status, and the availability, accessibility, acceptability, and utilization of health care services. Physical and social environmental factors include such things as air, water, housing, family structure, and funding changes.

3. *A sensor mechanism,* or some devised means for the continuous monitoring, identification, analysis, and feedforward of information on those external factors determined to be potentially disturbing to the agency's performance and the achievement of agency objectives. Feedforward of information differs from the feedback of information in that it is fed to appropriate staff in time for a direct assessment of disturbances in the system and corrective action before operations or outcomes are affected.

4. *The agency's internal operations (controlled input),* or those inputs over which the agency has control and is responsible and accountable. These inputs include resource allocation, structural characteristics, process activities, patient/family health outcomes (appropriate to achieving overall health and cost outcomes at the aggregate level) and measures of performance and accomplishments (predefined structure, process and outcome criteria and standards).

5. *Overall health and cost outcomes,* or what is actually accomplished in the target population at the aggregate level during care as measured by predefined criteria and standards.

6. *Feedforward and feedback of information on internal operations and actual health and cost outcomes,* or that data which are generated on a continuous basis through a built-in information system and are organized and interrelated to answer preformulated questions on the appropriateness of internal operations and the extent to which overall health and cost outcomes are achieved. Answers to questions are linked to an agency's planning, operational, evaluation, decision making, and reporting units. The ques-

tions themselves can be used to identify the data elements needed and thus avoid duplication of data collection.

7. *Agency administration,* or those persons who can effectively act to make the system perform as intended.

In order to establish how and whether an existing health care system is capable of delivering accessible, quality health care, it is useful to assess its current status within the context of these components. Following is a description of such an assessment in a hypothetical community health nursing agency prior to its use of the model.

A COMMUNITY HEALTH NURSING AGENCY BEFORE ITS USE OF THE MODEL

Figure 3 shows a hypothetical nursing agency prior to its use of the model. This agency is a large, voluntary organization that has been certified to serve Medicare and Medicaid patients. It serves an urban population of over 1.5 million and is characterized by all of the problems associated with such communities today.

Although I have selected one nursing agency for illustration purposes, Figure 3 is representative of many community health care agencies when viewed as a system within the context of the components described above.

As shown in Figure 3, this agency has developed written statements of philosophy, purpose, and policies. In fact, its stated purpose is to improve the health of the community it serves at an affordable cost. However, its statements of overall objectives are formulated as either broad activities or in general, vague, and unmeasureable terms rather than in expected health and cost outcomes for a target population. Therefore, objectives are not shown in Figure 3, only philosophy, purpose, and policies.

This agency also collected an enormous amount of information on the personal and environmental characteristics of the community, including information on the number, type, and use of its human service resources. Although this information is used by the agency to assess community needs, it is not used purposefully and explicitly as the basis and support for establishing a system capable of providing accessible, quality health care and achieving desired health and cost outcomes.

Instead, the data collected on the community as a whole are used by the agency primarily to document support for special budget requests, provide background information for special reports and proposals for funds, or to satisfy requests for information from myriad sources. In addition, this agency, like many, has no mechanism for identifying, monitoring, and counteracting those external factors that are likely to have a negative influence on its performance and/or accomplishments. Therefore, Figure 3 recognizes the existence of external constraints or factors, but they are not identified

FIGURE 3
Illustration of a Community Health Care Agency Prior to Its Use of a Modified System Control Model for Evaluation

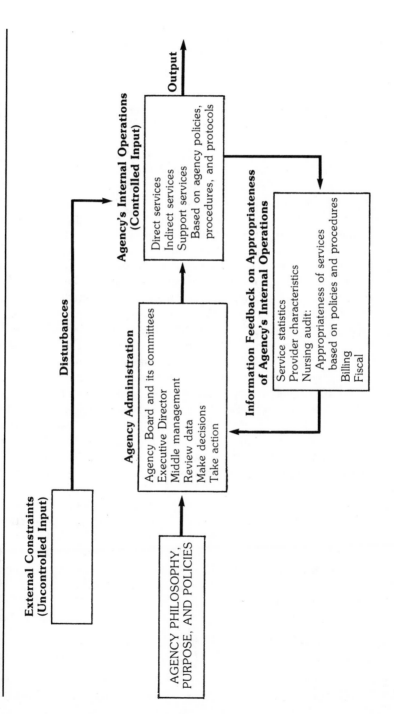

specifically for purposes of monitoring and counteracting their potentially disturbing effects. For this reason, these factors are shown dumping directly into the agency's internal operations, with no mechanism for analyzing and evaluating their impact on performance or the achievement of objectives.

In Figure 3, under internal operations, this agency is shown as having structured its services into direct, indirect, and support services. However, appropriateness of the activities, within each of the service components is based only on agency policies, procedures and protocols. Criteria and standards of practice or appropriate structure, process, and patient/family outcome have not been established.

Also in Figure 3, statements of actual overall health and cost outcomes are not shown for comparison with statements of desired health and cost objectives, because this agency has not established measureable health and cost objectives or outcomes. Therefore, only information on outputs or activities are depicted as being fed back to the agency's administrative and middle-management staffs in the form of service statistics (including some consumer characteristics), provider characteristics, billing and fiscal information, and the appropriateness of services based on agency policies and procedures. These data, of course, are not designed to answer questions on the extent to which the agency is providing accessible, quality health care or achieving desired health and cost outcomes in a target population.

As just described, this agency does not have measureable objectives nor a mechanism for identifying, monitoring, and counteracting external factors which could disturb the agency's performance. Nor does it have structure, process and outcome criteria and standards to guide professional practice and measure quality (appropriate structure, process, and patient/family outcomes). Consequently, it is not able to acquire concrete evidence of the extent to which it is providing quality care and achieving health outcomes. In the absence of such evidence, the agency does not have hard data to support such decisions as resource allocation and utilization—at least not with a high level of confidence that these changes can be expected to improve services and the health of people.

Since this agency is committed to an organized community effort to improve the health of the community as a whole as well as the population it serves, and since it is also being pressured for information that its current data base cannot provide, the evaluation committee was charged with responsibility for correcting agency deficiencies and establishing a system of health care services capable of delivering accessible, quality health care and achieving desired health and cost objectives.

A COMMUNITY HEALTH CARE AGENCY AFTER ITS USE OF THE MODIFIED MODEL

Figure 4 illustrates one of the agency's systems of services to a target population which the evaluation committee developed to correct the defi-

FIGURE 4
Illustration of a Community Health Care Agency Following its Use of a Modified System Control Model for Evaluation

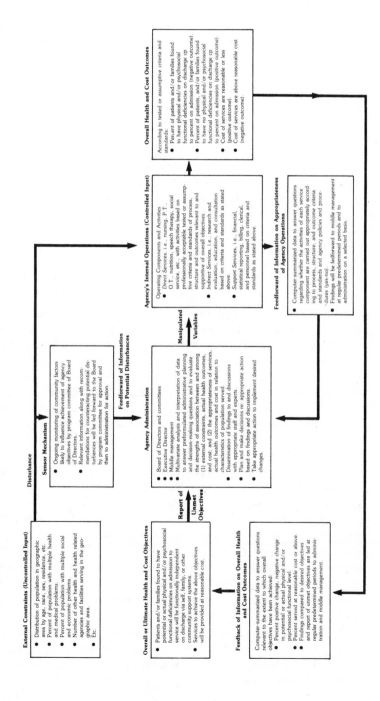

ciencies found during assessment. In the course of establishing this system, the evaluation committee asked and answered many questions. Some of them are shown in Figure 2. These sets of questions, among others, served to guide planning and corrective action and to achieve and maintain consistent inter-relationships between and among the components of the system.

For example, the agency in Figure 3 did not have measurable objectives based on identified community needs. Nor was it certain that its statements of community needs and agency philosophy, purpose, policies, and objectives were consistent in their interrelationships. Therefore, before this agency could formulate measurable health and cost objectives, all of its statements were reviewed to ensure completeness and consistency.

This review process began with a reassessment of selected, published data and general information on those personal and environmental characteristics of the community that are considered by recognized authorities as likely to contribute to or to interfere with health and health care. As a result of this reassessment, the evaluation committee found a number of changes since its last assessment.

For example, there had been a marked increase in the distribution of the population for the groups aged 5 to 19 and 65 or over. The distribution of the white and black populations also differed considerably, with the median age of the black population falling between 23 and 25, compared to 35 for the white population. The proportion of the population in the two lowest age groups (0-5 and 6-15) was about 50 percent higher among blacks than among whites. By contrast, the proportion of the population 65 years of age or over was more than twice as large among whites as among blacks.

The committee also found large pockets of sociopathology concentrated in three of the agency's six districts. These areas were characterized by low incomes, high unemployment, poor transportation, poor housing, low educational achievement levels, drug addiction, alcoholism, adolescent suicide, increased rates of teenage pregnancy, prematurity, and infant mortality.

In reviewing health care resources, the committee found a significant decrease in the number of private physicians serving these three districts but an equally significant increase in the number of private, ambulatory health care facilities, boarding homes, and nursing homes. However, there were no physicians available for housecalls. The newer type of health care facilities served special segments of the population who were either able to pay or were covered by some form of health insurance. In addition, the local health department had changed its practice of providing preventive services based on an assessment of the overall needs of the community. Although it was providing ambulatory family clinic services, there was no plan for identifying those individuals or segments of the population who could be characterized as vulnerable or at a high risk of illness but were not under care. Consequently, there was no plan for, or emphasis given to, outreach and early case finding, diagnosis, and treatment.

Along with the assessment of health problems and health care resources, the committee also assessed the community's strengths in terms of its ability to deal with its health and health-related problems. This assessment was based on documented utilization patterns, health care expenditures, and the findings of surveys concerned with the community's perception of the availability, accessibility, and acceptability of health care services.

Through a broad spectrum of such information as this, the evaluation committee was able to make a general assessment of the unmet health and health care needs of the community as a whole. These needs were used as the basis for reviewing, revising, or developing, as needed, all of the agency's statements of need, philosophy, purpose, policies, and objectives to reflect consistent interrelationships.

With the revised statements as a guide for establishing a system of services capable of delivering accessible, quality health care and achieving desired health and cost outcomes and with the components of the model as a framework for identifying, organizing, and interrelating numerous variables, the evaluation committee was able to use the questions in Figure 2 to develop an operational, measurable plan for correcting the deficiencies in one system of services. The committee was also able to build in an information system using data that were organized and interrelated to answer preformulated questions relevant to administrative, planning, evaluation, decision making and action. Following is a brief description of the plan.

Overall Health and Cost Objectives

Figure 4 shows that this agency has corrected its deficiencies and has established a system of health care services which it believes is capable of achieving its stated health and cost objectives. The plan has also been confirmed by a panel of experts which included both providers and consumers representative of a wide range of knowledge and skills.

Of the two objectives shown in Figure 4, one is concerned with health status and one with cost. The health objective is concerned with providing accessible, quality health care to patients/families then found to have potential or actual physical and/or psychosocial functional deficiencies on admission to service and with achieving functional independence by the time of discharge. Efforts to meet this objective will involve patients and their families or other community support systems. The cost objective is concerned with providing the service necessary to achieve the health objective at a reasonable cost.

These objectives were selected for the following reasons:

- They are congruent with identified, unmet needs of the community and with the broad goals of community health practice and the private medical community.

- They reflect the agency's belief in: (a) the uniqueness, wholeness, and unity of individuals in interaction with their physical and social environment; (b) health as a state of "wholeness"; (c) quality health care on a continuum at all levels of prevention, with a focus on the community as a whole; and (d) nursing as a process involving activities contributing to health, recovery, or peaceful death, which are carried out in a way that promotes maximum independence of the individual, the family, and the community.

- They are compatible with the responsibilities and functions of all agency personnel in the sense that all activities will be directed explicitly toward the achievement of both health and cost objectives.

- They are consistent with the current emphasis on the achievement and maintenance of physical and psychosocial functional independence as an ultimate, realistic goal of health care rather than simply the absence of disease.

- They parallel the current public concern with prevention, accessible quality health care, continuity of care, and cost containment.

- They are consistent with the goals of communities, families, and individuals who are concerned with how they will manage "when all the health workers have left the arena."

- The literature search indicated that there are reliable measures of physical functional and psychosocial health status and reasonable cost, and it seemed possible to describe other objectives in concrete, discernible criterion measures that could be tested for reliability.

External Constraints (Uncontrolled Input)

As used in this operational plan, external constraints are defined as those personal and environmental factors that are considered by recognized authorities as capable of influencing health, agency performance, and the achievement of health and cost objectives in a positive or negative way under certain circumstances. A few are shown in Figure 4. Other factors were described earlier and will not be repeated here.

Sensor Mechanism

Since these external factors can have a negative influence, it is essential that they be monitored, identified, and counteracted before they affect the agency's performance and the achievement of objectives. As shown in Figure 4, this agency has developed a strategy whereby the Program Committee of the Board will identify, analyze, and monitor these factors on a continuous basis. In addition, timely and relevant information on these factors, along with recommendations for action to counteract their potentially negative impact, will be fed forward to administration for implementation after approval by the Board. The Board and Program Committee are composed of members of the community who are representative of both providers and consumers with a wide variety of expertise. The Executive Director works closely with the Board and represents the input of agency staff into Board and committee deliberations.

Although the Program Committee will carry responsibility for monitoring external factors, there will be considerable interaction between and among the committee, the Board, and the Executive Director.

Agency's Internal Operation

As shown in Figure 4, this agency elected to retain the same three operating components that it had prior to the assessment. However, the activities of each operating component will be based on structure, process, and outcome criteria and standards appropriate for achieving desired health and cost outcomes. These criteria and standards will be collected or developed by staff representing all professional disciplines and other decision-making units. Criteria and standards of professional practice will be tested for reliability and validity.

Overall Health and Cost Outcomes

Measures of functional health outcomes will be collected or developed and tested for reliability and validity. Cost outcomes will be measured by regional or local criteria and standards of reasonable cost.

Feedback of Information

As shown in Figure 4, this agency will collect data to answer questions regarding whether the actitivies of each service component are carried out appropriately according to predefined structure, process, and outcome criteria and standards and agency policies and procedures. It will also collect data to answer questions on the extent to which overall objectives have been achieved. These data will be interrelated with data on the characteristics of the target population and fed back to administration and middle management at regular, predetermined periods for analysis, interpretation, dissemination, discussion of findings, and appropriate action.

The specific questions to be answered were formulated thoughtfully during the planning process at all levels of decision making. For example, on the administrative level, this agency formulated questions to acquire the information and evidence needed to: (1) demonstrate its ability to deliver accessible, quality health care and achieve predefined health and cost outcomes in target populations; (2) provide the basis for improving administrative planning, evaluation, decision making, and action in operational health care settings; and (3) meet its internal and external reporting requirements without duplicating data collection. Examples of these questions are as follows:

- What are the characteristics of the population served in relation to the characteristics of the target population?
- What happens to the health status of the population served during care?
- What agency resources are utilized to achieve what health and cost outcomes in the population served?
- What factors (internal and external) seem to be associated most consistently with what health and cost outcomes in the population served?

The formulation of these questions was guided by other questions. For example, what does an administrator of a community health care agency need to know about performance and accomplishments, and why? How will the information be used in planning, decision making and action? What data are needed? Can the data be practically and reliably collected? If so, how and from what source? Are valid and reliable criteria and standards available? If not can they be developed? How will the data be processed for analysis? How will the results be interpreted for planning, evaluation, decision making, and action?

Not until these questions were answered and data collection was considered feasible did the agency call in a computer vendor for consultation on the collection of data elements, forms design, data processing, and so forth. As a result, consultation was for more productive because the agency was clear about its objectives and the questions that needed to be answered.

Although not shown in this particular illustration, agency staff at all levels of decision making, including those in each operational component, participated in the formulation of questions relevant to their level of planning, evaluation, and decision making. Representatives of all professional disciplines also participated in the development of criteria and standards of practice. For this reason, every member of the staff is oriented thoroughly to the agency's overall objectives and its operational plan for achieving them.

Agency Administration

This agency's administration consists of the Board of Directors, the Executive Director, and middle-management staff. However, the Board and

Executive Director are ultimately responsible for assuring that the agency meets its overall objectives. They are also responsible for analyzing the factors associated with meeting objectives and the failure to meet objectives. As indicated in Figure 4, the action taken will be based on the analysis and interpretation of all data and the multivariate analysis of data on the agency's internal operation.

Now that this agency is organized purposefully and explicitly as a total system with a built-in method for generating data to answer preformulated questions, subsequent planning, evaluation, and decision making will be based on those factors (internal and external) which seem to be associated most consistently with favorable health and cost outcomes. As a result, decision makers at all levels in the organization will no longer have to tinker blindly with the interacting parts of the agency's operation.

But more important than any other use, the model provides a way for community health workers at all levels to communicate with each other within a common framework and to discover relationships between and among agency objectives, structural characteristics, process activities and patient/family outcomes at the individual and aggregate levels. As a result, planning, monitoring, evaluation, decision making, and action take on a new meaning to show what accessible, quality health care is and the difference it can make in the health of people. Now the consumers and purchasers of health care services can expect to receive credible answers to the questions of whether they are getting quality care for their health care dollars, how much it costs, and what good it is doing.

ABOUT THE AUTHOR

Mabel H. Morris, MA, RN, is retired and an independent consultant in Philadelphia, Pennsylvania. At the time this article was originally published, she was Nurse Consultant, Nursing Practice Branch, Division of Nursing, U.S. Department of Health, Education, and Welfare, Hyattsville, Maryland.

REFERENCES

1. H. C. Schulbert, A. Sheldon, and F. Baker, eds., *Program Evaluation in the Health Fields* (New York: Behavioral Publications, 1969).
2. R. Zemach, "Program Evaluation and System Control," *American Journal of Public Health,* 63 (July 1973), 607-609.

Data Utilization—for Successful Planning and Evaluation

Mary Lou Steedley

As discussed in the following piece, the Accreditation Program for Home Care and Community Health of the National League for Nursing has always been premised upon measurable program objectives stated in terms of client outcome. Steedley's article, published in 1979, remains useful today as a reference to assist agencies to focus on client outcomes. The article provides specific examples of program goals, measurable objectives stated in terms of client outcomes, and agency activities which support objectives in a method that incorporates accountability for evaluation. Several methods of data utilization are described for successful planning, care delivery, and evaluation in a community health agency. Each stresses the importance of participation by all agency staff.

A community health agency must develop a system that will provide the data needed for agency planning and evaluation if the agency is to function effectively and efficiently in providing services to its client population. We are all busy collecting data. We may even be drowning in data, but what

Reprinted from *Community Health: Today and Tomorrow,* copyright © 1979, National League for Nursing, New York, pp. 67-77.

is the result? Do we know the end product we seek? We are besieged by statistical requirements for our programs for funding and reimbursement; beside federal data requirements, there may be additional state requirements. We know what happened with the advent of Medicare, and even more statistics may be required if national health insurance becomes a reality.

Data collection systems should strive to obtain the necessary information as concisely, economically, and efficiently as possible. Data utilization is a tool—it can be a very effective tool—but is not an end in itself. To begin with, the agency must have a clear idea of the *objectives* of its data collection and of how the data will be utilized to reach them. A main objective of data collection should be to provide decision-makers at all levels with information relative to the agency's current activities, the results of these activities, and the extent to which the program objectives are being met. These data must then be useful for ongoing planning, both short-range and long-range.

Data can be utilized in three major ways:

1. Planning—to help determine what should be done and how to do it.
2. Control—the agency can keep statistical reports by employee in order to analyze activity by number of visits, type of visit, average time per visit, dollars of revenue, and related costs. Revenue and service reports can be obtained by discipline in order to evaluate the fees for a professional service.
3. Evaluation—the evaluation will tell how well the agency performed for a specific time period. Criteria must be developed against which to measure performance.

On a broader scope, home health agencies state that through the services provided certain community needs are met, cost of care is reduced when the patient is treated in his home environment, and the patient is able to recuperate more rapidly in the home/family environment. It is also claimed that the care provided is of high quality, that the multidisciplinary approach is most beneficial to the recipient of service, and that the delivery of services is provided in an appropriate, adequate, effective, and efficient manner. We speak of treating the whole individual and the value of continuity of patient care as the individual moves through different environments in the health care system. These statements certainly sound impressive, but more hard data are needed to substantiate these claims. More efforts need to be expended on obtaining hard data, not only within an agency but also based on a large population of agencies.

As we consider the activities within an individual agency, I will share with you the specifics of the system that was developed at Home Health Services of Louisiana, Inc., in 1976-1977. Special credit for the development of this system goes to Dr. Louis E. Barrilleaux, associate professor and director,

Middle-Management Center, Tulane University Center for Education, who served as a consultant, and the Professional Services Administration, including myself as director of professional services and Thania Elliot and Dorothy Thomas as associate directors of professional services. The direct services staff and supervisory staff of the agency were all involved in the process of the development of this system.

Within the agency, goals and objectives must be established. The *goals* may be established from two aspects—formative goals and summative goals—as was done at this agency. *Formative goals* are those that address the development and maintenance of an organizational capability as a prerequisite for providing quality patient care. From these, objectives can be formulated which improve organizational health. *Summative goals* are those that are directly related to the delivery of care, meeting the health needs of the community.

Below are the specific formative and summative goals developed at the agency in question:

Formative Goals

1. To provide communication linkages with the physicians, health and welfare agencies, and the aged residents of the community to enhance effective utilization of home health services.

2. To provide an agency environment which stimulates increased employee competence and job satisfaction for the delivery of high-quality service.

3. To provide community health learning experience for students at the undergraduate and graduate levels in the health and health-related fields.

Summative Goals

4. To provide a high-quality, comprehensive health care service through a coordinated plan of treatment to the chronically ill, aged, and disabled residents of the community.

5. To provide continuity of health care services in the referral mechanism in order to facilitate uninterrupted care for the individual patient within the health care system.

6. To provide the psychological and rehabilitative stimuli in order to promote recovery or the maximum rehabilitation of the individual in the home environment.

7. To provide appropriate environmental change in those situations when such action is indicated for the promotion and maintenance of health of the individual and his family.

From these goals, objectives are established for each agency program. The National League for Nursing conducts a program of accreditation for home health agencies and community nursing services, for which program they have established a number of criteria and a set of definitions to assist agencies in meeting those criteria. To define *program* and *objective,* I would like to quote their definitions:

> **Program**—A program is an organized agency response directed toward satisfying a community health need (or resolving a community health problem). Included in this response are stated objectives, performed activities, and utilized resources. Programs can be of varied scope and complexity. (*Examples:* maternal child health program, communicable disease control program, care of sick program (home health), school health program, etc.)
>
> **Program Objective**—An objective is an expected or desired outcome. It specifies what one wishes to accomplish. It is expressed in terms that can be measured. *Examples:*
>
> **Care of Sick Program:**
> *Objective:* 80 percent of the total patients with diagnosed illnesses will be able to maintain themselves independently or with family assistance within a three-month period of admission to the program.
>
> **MCH Program:**
> *Objective:* 50 percent of the pregnant teenagers within the Central City district will understand the importance and be under medical supervision before the fifth month of pregnancy.[1]

The agency's program objectives are contained in its summative goals. The objectives are all patient-related in behavioral terms and are measurable. In Figure 1, we have an example from the Home Health Services of Louisiana, Inc., of the translation of a specific goal (in this case a summative one) into definite program objective (left-hand column).

After the agency has developed its goals and program objectives, it must then develop *process objectives,* which are the methods to be used and the actions to be taken to meet the program objectives. Referring again to the NLN-APHA criteria and definitions, we find *activities* defined as follows:

> **Activities**—Activities are defined as the methods used and/or actions taken to accomplish the program objectives. *Examples:*
>
> **Care of Sick Program:**
> *Activities:* Nurse makes home visits and
> • *Assesses* patient and family.
> • *Gives* direct care.
> • *Demonstrates* procedures.
> • *Teaches* patient/family members, etc.
>
> **MCH Program:**
> *Activities:* Establishes maternity clinic for teenagers in Central City area. The nurse

- *Disseminates information* concerning health facilities available.
- *Interprets* need for adequate health supervison.
- *Teaches* physical change and continual effects of normal pregnancy, etc.[2]

In the second column of Figure 1 are examples of the translation of the program objectives into *process objectives* or *activities.*

The next big step is program evaluation. The design for this evaluation involves looking at each specific program objective. This step includes the utilization of assessment or monitoring tools to substantiate the extent to which the objectives have been reached. These tools may include such things as clinical records, utilization review committee records, nursing audit forms, case conference records, records of the periodic review of patient progress committee, personnel records, performance evaluations, interagency memos, schedules, staff meeting reports or minutes, patient discharge forms, Professional Advisory Committee reports or minutes, reports or minutes from meetings of the Board of Directors, or any other agency reports or records that might contain data helpful in assessing and monitoring the activity.

Figure 2 shows a sample evaluation of goal IV and program objective IV-A. The first column lists the *indicators,* which are the specific patient outcomes. The next column shows the data sources from which you expect to provide evidence of your activity in meeting the objective. And the third column shows the findings of your examination of the data.

The total evaluation design does not end here, however. Now that the agency has the findings, they must be shared with appropriate administrative and service personnel. It is important to get the service staff's reaction to the findings. What are the recommendations from the findings and staff feedback? The decisions made on such feedback and recommendations should involve the service staff and administration. If the program objective was not met, review the process objectives (activities) to assess the extent to which they were carried out. Also, assess whether the program objective is realistic or needs revision.

The next step is the action taken based on the findings and recommendations from staff and others. Then the process begins again; evaluation is an ongoing process.

To review, the agency identifies goals, program objectives, process objectives (activities), and assessment and monitoring tools for ongoing operation and knowledge of the desired end result. The evaluation design, as developed by Home Health Services of Louisiana and as shown in Figure 3, involves:

1. Program objectives—Specific program objectives.

2. Indicators—Specific patient outcomes.

3. Data sources—Identified data sources.

FIGURE 1
Agency Goal Translated into Program Objectives

Goal IV. To provide a high quality comprehensive health care service through a coordinated plan of treatment to the chronically ill, aged, and disabled residents of the community.

Program Objectives	Process Objectives (Activities)	Assessment / Monitoring
IV-A. Given a three-month admission period to the program, at least 50% of patients with *acute* illnesses will recover their health and demonstrate actions which will promote optimum health.	IV-1. **Service:** This category of activities refers to *all* professional personnel who visit patients in their homes to:	
	IV-1.1. Assess patients and family needs.	IV-1.1M. Clinical record, Utilization Review Committee form, Nursing Audit Report Form.
IV-B. Given a four-month admission period to the program, at least 45% of patients with *chronic* illnesses will achieve maximum recovery within the defined limits of their diseases or disabilities.	IV-1.2. Give patient care, including treatments and preventive procedures requiring substantial specialized skills.	IV-1.2M. Clinical record, supervisory field visits as documented in personnel records.
	IV-1.3. Teach, supervise, and counsel the patient and family regarding the health care needs and other related problems of the patient.	IV-1.3M. Clinical record, supervisory field visits as documented in personnel records, Utilization Review Committee form, Nursing Audit Report form.
IV-C. At least 50% of patients in the *terminal* stage of their illness and/or their families will demonstrate the ability to cope with the emotional and physical aspects of a terminal disease, as evidenced by less pain and fear, and by increased ability to handle crisis.	IV-1.4. Observe signs and symptoms of reactions to treatments and drugs and changes in patient's physical and emotional condition and report and consult with patient's physician as frequently as needed.	IV-1.4M. Clinical record, reports to supervisor, Utilization Review Committee form, Nursing Audit Report form.
	IV-1.5. Assist patients and/or families to utilize appropriate community resources.	IV-1.5M. Clinical record, medical social work referrals, Utilization Review and Patient Progress Committee forms.

FIG. 1 (continued)

Program Objectives	Process Objectives (Activities)	Assessment / Monitoring
	IV-1.6. Provide emotional support and/or counsel with the terminally ill patient and/or his family.	IV-1.6M. Clinical record.
	IV-1.7. The home health aide provides a distinct contribution in the coordinated treatment plan by direct assistance and care to patients as instructed by the professional staff.	IV-1.7M. Clinical record, home health aide assignment form.
	IV-2. Support: *All* professional personnel perform the following supportive activities to enhance the delivery of direct patient care:	
	IV-2.1. Establish patient goals and develop a plan of care with the needs and well-being of the patient as the central focus and in accordance with the physician's.	IV-2.1M. Clinical record, Utilization Review Committee form, Nursing Audit Report form, Periodic Review of Patient Progress Committee form.
	IV-2.2. Establish and maintain an accurate clinical record.	IV-2.2M. Clinical record, Nursing Audit Report form, Utilization Review Committee form, Supervisor Record Review form.
	IV-2.3. Coordinate total patient care by communication with other team members, health providers, and community resources when indicated.	IV-2.3M. Clinical record, referral forms, Periodic Review of Patient Progress Committee form, Utilization Review Committee form, reports to Supervisor.

FIG. 1 (continued)

Program Objectives	Process Objectives (Activities)	Assessment / Monitoring
	IV-2.4. Supervise and instruct the home health aide in patient care activities.	IV-2.4M. Clinical record, Home Health Aide Evaluations, reports to Home Health Aide Supervisor, Anecdotal notes.
	IV-3. **Administration:** The following administrative activities are performed to facilitate both direct and supportive quality patient care:	
	IV-3.1. The associate directors of professional services recruit, orient, and maintain qualified nursing, occupational therapy, nutrition, and medical social service personnel according to agency policies and state and national requirements for professional personnel to meet service projections of all eligible patients.	IV-3.1M. Personnel records, reports to administration and board, weekly and monthly activity reports, orientation outline.
	IV-3.2. The physical therapy and speech pathology supervisors recruit, orient, and maintain qualified therapy personnel according to agency policies and state and national requirements for professional personnel to meet service projections of all eligible patients.	IV-3.2M. Personnel records, reports to administration and board, weekly and monthly activity reports, orientation outline.
	IV-3.3. The associate directors of professional services, associate director for administration, and supervisors provide adequate supervision to their respective personnel through orientation, reporting, on-site field visits, and conferences.	

Developed by Home Health Services of Louisiana management staff. Used by permission.

4. Findings—The findings reported in narrative or table format.

5. Feedback suggestions—Staff reaction to the findings.

6. Recommendations—Recommendations resulting from the findings and feedback.

7. Action taken—Identified actions taken based on the recommendations.

Agencies are accountable for their operations. To assist them with this accountability, systems should be in effect or should be developed that will provide: (1) a method for the evaluation of the direct patient care provided (quality assurance mechanisms); (2) data about the amount and type of service provided; (3) data concerning the outcome (results) of the service; and (4) an evaluation mechanism for total agency operation.

Management information systems are being used by many agencies to assist in obtaining data. When looking at your management information system or exploring the field for utilization, consider:

1. The type of information the system generates. Will it be useful to your agency? Will it meet your needs?

2. The cost of utilizing the system. Will the agency realize savings by using the system instead of collecting data manually? What is included in the cost? Does the cost cover input and output documents or does it include services such as mailing, training of agency staff, consultation to the agency for input problems, correcting input problems, etc.?

3. The accuracy and timeliness of receiving the data.

4. Will the system make changes as needed; will it expand and remain current with the field?

There are several management information systems available to home health agencies. As an example, I would like to list a sample few of the output documents that are produced by the management information system utilized by Unihealth Services Corporation:

• Patient ledger with visit and fee register.

• Number of patients and visits by diagnosis and service.

• Number of discharged patients and visits by discharge reason and type of service.

• Agency employee utilization.

• Number of patients by area code and diagnosis.

I have discussed several methods of data utilization for successful planning and evaluation. Data utilization is a tool, and can be a very effective tool, to assist with agency planning, delivery of care, and the evaluation

FIGURE 2
Sample Evaluation of Goal and Program Objectives

Goal IV. To provide a high quality comprehensive health care service through a coordinated plan of treatment to the chronically ill, aged, and disabled residents of the community.

Program Objective IV-A. Given a three-month admission period to the program, at least 50 percent of patients with acute illnesses will recover their health and demonstrate actions which will promote optimum health.

Indicators	Data Source	Findings
Discharge category of "maximum rehabilitation" was indicative of patients recovering their health. Patients with primary admission diagnosis in the following categories were grouped into *acute illnesses:* 1. Infective and parasitic diseases. 2. Neoplasms with surgical procedures but without metastases. 3. Diseases of the circulatory system (pulmonary emboli and acute congestive heart failure only). 4. Diseases of the digestive system. 5. Urinary tract infections. 6. Diseases of the skin and subcutaneous tissue, including decubitus ulcers. 7. Accidents, poisoning, and violence (nature of injury).	A 10% random sample of charts was selected from all patients admitted from June 1, 1975, to May 31, 1976. A total of 1,093 patients were admitted in fiscal year 1976. Every tenth chart was selected, based on a numerical list assigned by admitting department to all new patients. A total of 106 charts were reviewed.	1. Total number of patients: 38 2. Discharge reasons: Maximum rehabilitation—27 patients (71%) Institutionalized—11 patients (29%) 3. Length of service to reach maximum rehabilitation: *Month* *Patients* *Percentage* 0-1 4 11% 1-2 9 24% 2-3 7 18% 3-4 7 18% Total 27 71% 4. Within four months of admission to the program, 27 patients (71%) with *acute* illnesses had reached maximum rehabilitation. 5. Within three months of admission to the program, 20 patients (53%) with *acute* illnesses had reached maximum rehabilitation.

FIGURE 3
Evaluation Design

Program Objectives	Indicators	Data Sources	Findings		Feedback Suggestions	Recommenda-tions	Action Taken
List specific program objective.	Process objectives or activities. (Specific patient outcomes.)	What is specific data source?	What are findings? (Reported in narrative or table format.)		What are staff reactions to findings? Decision on action to be taken involves the entire staff.	What are recommenda-tions resulting from findings and staff feedback?	What actions occurred based on recommenda-tions?

process. In this process, you identify strengths and weaknesses. Where weakness is identified, the agency produces change. Where strengths are identified, the agency can validate its activities with hard data. Proper utilization of data is a tool to assist you in attaining your agency goals and program objectives, of which the major consideration in every agency must be to provide quality patient care as appropriately, adequately, economically, and efficiently as possible.

ABOUT THE AUTHOR

At the time of writing, Mary Lou Steedley was Vice President, Professional Services, Unihealth Services Corporation, New Orleans, Louisiana.

REFERENCES

1. National League for Nursing, Council of Home Health Agencies and Community Health Services, and American Public Health Association, *Accreditation of Home Health Agencies and Community Nursing Services: Criteria and Guide for Preparing Reports* (New York: National League for Nursing, 1976), 22–23.
2. Ibid.

Program Objectives

Visiting Nurse Association
of Metropolitan Atlanta

This excerpt is an example of one agency's approach to writing program objectives for its home health services. It provides a process format for consideration in the evaluation of agency programs.

HOME HEALTH SERVICES

Overall Objectives

To assist those in need of therapeutic treatment services to regain functioning, to become rehabilitated to the extent possible, and to achieve stability of their pathological condition.

To assist those with chronic illness and disability to remain in their homes as long as it is safe, comfortable, and medically and functionally feasible for them to do so.

Reprinted with permission of Visiting Nurse Association of Metropolitan Atlanta, Atlanta, Georgia.

Supporting Objectives

1. To improve the functioning status of 70 percent of the patients who were in need of therapeutic treatment and admitted for home health services.

2. To assist 70 percent of the patients who on admission have an expected outcome of "independent" in functioning status to become independent at time of discharge.

3. Within two months of admission either to discharge or reduce service requirements of 55 percent of the patients admitted.

4. To achieve 60 percent of the goals established for patients.

5. To have 90 percent of the records reviewed in utilization review show that services were integrated, that needs were met, and that there was an appropriate relationship between the care plan and services provided to the patient's condition and course of illness.

6. To assist those with a terminal illness to die at home as long as it is safe and within the patient's/family's physical and emotional capabilities.

7. To prevent exacerbation of illness and/or disability necessitating institutionalization in 75 percent of patients served.

Activities

The activities performed to achieve the objectives of the home health services program are divided into five major categories: assessment, establishment of a care plan, intervention, coordination, and evaluation.

Assessment.

1. Collect baseline data on patient's physical, social and environmental condition through interviews, examination, observation, and review of pertinent health records.

2. Conduct further in-depth assessment of specific needs identified as appropriate for physical, speech, or occupational therapy or medical social service.

Establishment of Care Plan.

1. Identify problems/needs that necessitate agency intervention.

2. Identify the goals and objectives of care in measurable terms.

3. Identify target dates for the accomplishment of each objective.

4. Develop a plan of actions/activities to be taken by all care providers, indicating treatment modalities and frequency of interventions.

5. Review care plan with the attending physician and obtain signed orders for the services to be provided by the agency.

Intervention.

1. Provide services consistent with the care plan.

2. Provide direct care.

3. Teach patient/family members to achieve independence in appropriate areas.

4. Supervise services provided by paraprofessionals.

5. Refer to other professional services within the agency and initiate referrals to appropriate community resources.

6. Document the care provided directly and activities performed on behalf of the patient in the case record.

Coordination.

1. Participate in weekly and monthly conferences with direct care providers to review the course of treatment and the patient's responsiveness to the care being provided.

2. As often as required/needed, review the activities of the homemaker/home health aide with the patient and family and document the aide's activities to be performed.

3. Review the documentation completed by the homemaker/home health aide and conduct joint visits to assure appropriate services.

4. Establish and maintain contacts, both formal and informal, with other community agencies serving the patient/family.

5. Communicate directly to the physician when there is a change in the patient's condition and provide a written summary of the patient's response to treatment at least every sixty days.

Evaluation.

1. Identify the results of the activities performed in providing care and the observed changes in the patient's condition.

2. Modify goals and activities for the patient's care as needed as a result of the evaluation.

3. Determine appropriate continuation of service.

Health Promotion and Disease Prevention Emphasis Plan

Oklahoma City Area Indian Health Service

These excerpts from the Health Promotion and Disease Prevention Emphasis Plan *were submitted to the National League for Nursing as part of a self-study for accreditation in the Home Care and Community Health Program. In it, the Oklahoma Indian Health Service provides an excellent example of program objectives stated in aggregate client outcome terms. The client is the focus, the desired result or behavior is specified, and time frames are identified with a quantifiable standard (percentage) against which results can be evaluated. This plan transforms "idealistic" public health goals into realistic and measurable program objectives in a fashion that will provide a positive evaluation for direct service staff as well as for the federal government.*

INTRODUCTION AND OVERVIEW OF PLAN

The Health Promotion/Disease Prevention programs have been called the second public health revolution. The first was the struggle against infectious diseases which spanned the late 19th century and the first half of the 20th century.

Reprinted with permission from *Health Promotion and Disease Prevention Plan*, Oklahoma City Area Indian Health Service, Oklahoma City, OK, June 1986.

Many programs sprang up throughout the nation aimed at health promotion and disease prevention, but the first national document which spoke directly to these areas was *Healthy People, the Surgeon General's Report on Health Promotion and Disease Prevention* which was published in 1979. Following this in 1980 the book *Promoting Health and Preventing Disease: Objectives for the Nation* was published.

The following plan was developed by several members of an area committee who consulted with health providers throughout the Oklahoma Area. The baseline data which is given comes from Oklahoma State Health Department Statistics, census reports, IHS statistics, and independent surveys. The plan is an attempt to condense the almost 300 objectives that are found in the book *Promoting Health and Preventing Disease: Objectives for the Nation.* The 15 areas in that book have been reassembled into the 12 you find in this plan in order to address more precisely the health problems and conditions in the Oklahoma Service Area.

GOALS AND OBJECTIVES

As you read the plan your first response may be that it is unrealistic and impossible to reach each one of the objectives within the stated time frames. Please stop and think that many of the process objectives are already in place, and that some of the goals have already been reached. The goals were written in the most idealistic of terms so that the optimum could be achieved, or at least attempted. It was felt that to lower the goals could be interpreted as attempting to achieve less than quality care for our people. So a balance had to be reached between striving for the impossible and setting goals so low that progress would not be achieved.

Each Service Area will be responsible for meeting the goals as stated in the plan unless they develop revised ones specific to their own area. Any specific goals should be measurable and should show a degree of progress. For example, one goal states there will be "a minimum of monthly contacts with 50 percent of overweight patients." It would be impossible for a large facility to accomplish this within their present resources. Therefore, a revised goal could be established that "50 patients who are 150 percent or more over their ideal weight will be counseled bimonthly over a one-year period with a goal of at least 20 percent weight loss for each person." Another example is how baseline data can be obtained. Until all computers are functioning and programs are written, complete baseline data is very difficult to obtain. Therefore, a Service Area could do a random chart audit of a certain number of records to determine their baseline.

I. Chronic Disease

Goal: *To reduce the complications and mortality from diabetes, hypertension, cardiovascular disease, and cancer.*

Data Base: OSHD Statistics for Indians
* Mortality 1984
  1. Diabetes—27.3/100,000
  2. Hypertension—8.3/100,000
  3. All cardiovascular disease—218.8/100,000
  4. Cancer—108.2/100,000

* Complication data—not complete
  1. Indians in Oklahoma with diabetic end-stage renal disease in 1984 = 64 (Source: Network X—End-Stage Renal Disease)
  2. Amputations performed in Oklahoma IHS hospitals in 1984 = 88

Outcome Objective 1
By the end of 1986 all facilities will have a system (i.e., problem list, computer program) for identifying and establishing a data base of the number of complications from chronic diseases. At a minimum to identify:

1. Diabetic retinopathy
2. Amputations from diabetes
3. Renal disease from diabetes and hypertension
4. Cardiac disability—i.e., inability to work, or carry out activities of daily living
5. Cancer which could and should have been diagnosed earlier

Outcome Objective 2
By the end of 1986 each Service Unit will have a community action plan in place for the primary and secondary prevention of chronic diseases.

1. The primary prevention plan will include:
   a. A minimum of monthly sessions in schools and/or the community regarding healthy behaviors such as the need for exercise, proper diet, avoidance of smoking and contact with toxic agents, reduction of stress, danger signs of cancer, etc.
   b. Establishment of systematic wellness services at each facility for patients.
   c. Establishment of wellness services in all employee health programs.

d. Anti-smoking campaigns at all facilities with 50 percent smoke-free by 1986, and 100 percent smoke-free by 1987.

2. The secondary prevention plan will include:
   a. Early screening for hypertension—by 1990, 90 percent of all patients over age 12 will have an annual BP recorded on their medical record.
   b. By 1990 all patients with a family history of diabetes, and 50 percent of patients exceeding their ideal body weight by 20 percent, will have annual random blood sugars.
   c. Early cancer detection—by 1990 all facilities will have systematic cancer screening services in place (see 1-7 for specifics).
   d. By 1990 all facilities will have a weight reduction program (for the "healthy obese") which includes changes in both diet and exercise.
   e. All facilities by 1990 will have available smoking cessation services for the "healthy smokers."
   f. All facilities by the end of 1986 will have a special emphasis plan for the prevention and control of gestational diabetes.

Outcome Objective 3

By 1990 the number of identified diabetics under adequate long-term control defined as a blood sugar of less than 150 mg for at least two years will increase by 5 percent annually.

Data Base: Number of diabetic patients and number under control—not available

Process Objectives:

1. By the end of 1987, there will be a system in place at all facilities to identify patients with diabetes, to identify those under control, and to recall those not under control for regular follow-up.
2. By 1990, 90 percent of all diabetic patients will have evidence of patient education documented a minimum of two times yearly which includes diet, exercise, foot care, smoking, hygiene, medication administration, danger signs of hypo- and hyperglycemia, and stress reduction.
3. By 1990, 90 percent of all diabetics will have evidence of a foot exam on each visit and an annual eye exam.

Outcome Objective 4

By 1990, 60 percent of all identified hypertensives will be under long-term adequate control as defined by BP of less than 140/90 for at least two years.

Data Base: Number of hypertensive patients and number under control—not available

Process Objectives:

1. By the end of 1987 there will be a system in place at all facilities to identify patients with hypertension, to identify those under control, and a method for recalling those not under control for regular follow-up.

2. By 1990, 90 percent of all hypertensive patients will have evidence of patient education a minimum of two times yearly which includes diet, exercise, foot care, smoking, and medication administration.

Outcome Objective 5

By 1990 the prevalence of significant obesity defined as 120 percent of desired weight will be reduced 20 percent for all age groups without nutritional impairment.

Data Base: Not available

Process Objectives:

1. By the end of 1986 all facilities will have a system in place to identify and establish a baseline of the target overweight population

2. By the end of 1986 all facilities will have a weight reduction program implemented which includes at minimum:
   a. Community and school education (ref. Obj. I-2)
   b. Self-help groups
   c. Diet history for all patients.
   d. Diet plan for all overweight patients
   e. Minimum of monthly contacts with 50 percent of overweight patients (target population to be set by each Service Area)

Outcome Objective 6

By 1990, the incidence of smoking will be reduced by 50 percent.

Data Base: Not available

Process Objectives:

1. By the end of 1986 all facilities will have a system (i.e., problem list) to identify and establish a baseline on the number of smokers at their facility.

2. By 1986, 50 percent of facilities will be smoke-free and by beginning 1987, 100 percent will be smoke-free.

3. Smoking prevention and cessation programs will be available at all facilities by the end of 1986.

4. By 1988, 90 percent of smokers will have documented evidence at each contact that smoking cessation has been discussed and a program has been offered.

Outcome Objective 7

By 1990 all facilities will have an ongoing early cancer detection and screening program.

Process Objectives:

1. By 1990, 90 percent of all patients over age 40 will have a hemnocult stool test annually.

2. By 1990, 90 percent of all women sexually active or over age 25 will have annual pap smear and breast exams.

3. By 1990, 90 percent of all women screened over the age of 20 will be taught how and why to do a self-breast exam.

4. By 1990, 90 percent of adults will have been given material explaining the seven danger signs of cancer.

5. By 1990, 90 percent of adult males (peak age is 15-25) will have been taught how and why to do a testicular exam.

6. By 1990, 90 percent of all males over the age of 50 will have a yearly exam for cancer of the prostate.

7. Anti-smoking campaigns will be conducted in all facilities and 50 percent will be smoke-free by 1986, and 100 percent by 1987.

II. Family Planning

Goal: *To reduce the number of unwanted pregnancies and to reduce the number of high-risk pregnancies by 25 percent by 1990.*

Data Base: Source: Oklahoma State Health Statistics
  • Unwanted pregnancies—Data not available
  • High-risk pregnancies—Complete data not available
    Deliveries to women under age 17 in 1984 = 464 (9.08 percent)
    Deliveries to women over age 35 in 1984 = 200 (4.02 percent)

Process Objectives:

1. By the end of 1986 there will be an Area standard definition of a high-risk pregnancy, and by 1987 there will be a system in place to identify the number of high-risk pregnancies.

2. By 1987 a system will be in place at all facilities to identify the number of unintended pregnancies.

3. By 1986 all facilities will have qualified staff designated, audiovisual material available, and a regular program in place to provide family planning information in the hospitals and clinics.

4. In each facility by the end of 1986 there will be documented evidence of family planning education in schools and/or the community at least on a quarterly basis.

5. By the end of 1986, 90 percent of all women of childbearing age and 100 percent of women in high-risk groups accessing Oklahoma facilities will have documented evidence that family planning services have been offered.

6. By 1987, 90 percent of postpartum patients requesting sterilization will have services provided immediately following delivery; 90 percent of all other patients (male and female) requesting sterilization will have services available within 30 days following the required waiting period.

III. Maternal Health

Goal: *To reduce or maintain the maternal mortality rate of less than 5 per 100,000 pregnancies.*

Data Base:
1984 Oklahoma rate = 0
1983 Oklahoma rate = 0.6 (1 case)
1982 Oklahoma rate = 0

Process Objectives:
1. Family planning services will be increased, especially to high-risk groups (ref: Goal II).

2. By the end of 1986, 90 percent of all women will begin prenatal care by the end of their second trimester. All prenatal clients will receive a special emphasis program on the prevention and/or control of gestational diabetes and the danger of alcohol consumption, substance abuse, and smoking during pregnancy.
   Data base: 1985, 87.9 percent of all women began their prenatal care by the end of the second trimester.

3. By the end of 1986, 60 percent of teens (under age 20) will begin prenatal care by the end of their first trimester.
   Data base: 1985, 56.6 percent of teens began their prenatal care by the end of the first trimester.

4. By 1990, 90 percent of all prenatal will have a minimum of 10 prenatal clinic visits, high-risk patients will have 12.
   Data base: Not determined at this time.

5. By 1990, 90 percent of all high-risk prenatal patients will be counseled and/or visited by community services (CHN, Social Service, Nutrition and Health Education) at least once during the pregnancy and as early as possible to determine needs.

6. By 1986, 90 percent of all prenatal patients will be referred to an obstetrician by the third visit, or 28th week, to assess risk category and pregnancy management.

IV. Infant Health

Goal: *By 1990, the neonatal mortality rate will not exceed 6.5 deaths per 1,000 live births; and the infant mortality rate will not exceed 9 per 1,000.*

Data Base: Oklahoma State Health Department Statistics for Indians
1982 neonatal rate = 4.8 infant rate = 8.6
1983 neonatal rate = 4.7 infant rate = 8.4
1984 neonatal rate = 3.7 infant rate = 6.7

Note: Since Oklahoma's Indian population statistics have reached the national goals, Oklahoma Indian Health Service goal will be to maintain or decrease those statistics by 1990.

Process Objectives:

1. Promote prenatal and family planning services (ref. Goals II, III).

2. By 1990, all facilities will have genetic counseling available.

3. By 1987, there will be a minimum of one level II nursery in Oklahoma Indian Health Service.

4. By 1990, all high-risk infants born in IHS hospitals will have access by direct referral to high-risk nursery care.

5. By the end of 1986 all IHS facilities will have a community awareness program directed toward the need for well child care.

6. By the end of 1986 all children born in IHS hospitals will be discharged with an infant car seat; and a program will be implemented to provide assistance to obtain car seats for Indian children not born in IHS hospitals.

7. By the end of 1986 all facilities will maintain high-risk infant registries, and 95 percent of these infants will receive well child services appropriate for age according to the American Academy of Pediatrics; and, 90 percent of non-high-risk infants will receive appropriate well child services. Well child services will include at

minimum growth and development, physical assessment, accident prevention counseling, dietary history with infant and child feeding counseling, recognition of the danger signs of infant illness, immunizations, and the need for infant stimulation (ref. IHS Maternal and Child Health Manual, Chapter 13).

V. Child Health

Goal: *By 1990, 90 percent of all children up through adolescence will receive appropriate health services and high-risk groups will be identified and given special services.*

Process Objectives:

1. By the end of 1986 all facilities will maintain a handicapped child registry. There will be an interdisciplinary committee which develops a plan of care for each child. Each child will be assigned a case manager who will present the plan and progress of the child as often as necessary but at least annually to the committee.

2. By the end of 1986 all facilities will have a Child Abuse/Neglect Committee which maintains a registry of all appropriate children and reviews each case as needed but at least annually.

3. By 1987, all facilities will establish, or have available adolescent health care clinics which include psychosocial services.

4. By 1990, 90 percent of all children will continue well child care throughout childhood as recommended by the American Academy of Pediatrics (12 months, 18 months, 2 years, 3, 5-6, 8-9, 11-12, 13-15, 16-20). Special attention to be given to diet, prevention of teenage pregnancy, emotional health, prevention of substance abuse, and accident prevention since it is the leading cause of death for children.

VI. Immunization

Goal: *To prevent or decrease the incidence of vaccine-preventable diseases.*

Data Base: 1985 Oklahoma State Health Department Statistics for Indians
Diphtheria, tetanus—No cases reported
Pertussis—8 cases reported
Measles—No cases reported
Mumps—No cases reported

Rubella—No cases reported
Hepatitis B—15 cases reported
Influenza—No data reported
Pneumococcal disease—No data reported
H influenza—20 cases reported (5 over age 24 months)

Process Objectives:

1. By the end of 1986 all facilities will have a system in place to identify and track patients and their immunization status.

2. By 1986 all facilities will have a community awareness program directed toward the need for immunizations for both children and adults. (Evidence of quarterly emphasis programs; i.e., prenatal classes, school programs, elder care programs, media coverage, etc.)

3. By the end of 1986, 90 percent of all children under the age of 27 months will be appropriately immunized for age for DPT, MMR, polio, and H influenza.

4. By 1986, 90 percent of adolescents will have boosters for Td.

5. By 1990, 60 percent of targeted adults will have appropriate immunizations for Td, MMR, hepatitis B, influenza, and pneumococcal disease.

6. By 1987, all facilities will have employee health programs which insure all employees have been immunized against rubella or have a positive titer, and all high-risk employees have been immunized for hepatitis B and influenza.

VII. Communicable Diseases, Including Sexually Transmitted Diseases

Goal: *To reduce or prevent the incidence of infectious and communicable diseases, not controlled by vaccines.*

Data Base:

Tuberculosis—National objective 8/100,000 rate
Oklahoma 1984 rate = 26.7/100,000 (45 cases)

Hepatitis A—No national objective
Oklahoma 1984 rate = 41.6/100,000 (70 cases)

Salmonellosis—No national objective
Oklahoma 1984 rate = 118/100,000 (20 cases)

Shigellasis—No national objective
Oklahoma 1984 rate = 10.1/100,000 (17 cases)

Gonorrhea—National objective 280/100,000
Oklahoma 1984 rate = 288/100,000 (485 cases)

Syphilis—National objective 7/100,000
Oklahoma 1984 rate = 7.7/100,000 (13 cases)

Nosocomial Infections—National average = 3.5/100 discharges
Oklahoma rate = 2.6/100 discharges

AIDS—No national objective
Oklahoma rate 1984 = no cases

Process Objectives:

1. By the end of 1986 all facilities should have a community awareness and education program directed toward the prevention and early recognition of communicable diseases. Emphasis on STD in the adolescent and young adult group.
2. By 1986, all facilities should have a registry of TB patients and should review cases on a quarterly basis with the county/or state health department.
3. Protocols should be in place at all facilities by 1986 for the recognition, reporting, contact investigation, and treatment of all communicable diseases, including STD.
4. All hospitals should continue their infection control programs and all health centers should have developed and implemented an infection control program by end of 1986.
5. Community education programs should be held quarterly on proper sanitation, hygiene, and food preparation needed to prevent and control communicable diseases.

VIII. Dental Health

Goal: *To reduce the prevalence of dental caries and disease.*

Data Base:

1. 1985—50 percent of preschoolers in Oklahoma had nursing bottle caries
   Outcome objective in 1990 = reduce to 25 percent
2. 1985 estimate of unmet dental needs in categories 1-3 (emergency, preventive, and routine restorative) = 36 percent
   Outcome objective in 1990 = reduce to 25 percent

Process Objectives:

1. By 1990, increase the number of clients served by community flouridation systems to 75 percent.
   Data 1985: 50 percent.

2. By 1988 all facilities will have a system in place to identify children not served by fluoridated water systems and to monitor dietary fluoride supplementation.

3. By 1990, 75 percent of children under age 20 not served by community fluoridated systems will be receiving dietary fluoride supplements and oral hygiene and dietary counseling.

4. By 1990, 90 percent of new mothers will receive education on the cause and prevention of nursing bottle caries.

5. By 1990, 90 percent of all aged patients will be receiving education regarding dental health.

6. By 1986, all IHS dental programs will offer each dental patient individualized prevention planning services to include fluoride, pit and fissue sealants, oral hygiene instruction, and dietary counseling.

IX. Substance Abuse

Goal: *To reduce morbidity and mortality associated with substance abuse.*

Data Base:

1. Number of children born with recognized FAS in Oklahoma in 1985 = 0

2. Mortality from cirrhosis and chronic liver disease in 1984 = 29 cases; 17.2 rate (OSHD statistics)

3. Number OPVs for substance abuse related accidents with injuries in 1985 = 865; total accidents = 17,330 (IHS program data)

4. Number of motor vehicle accidents and mortality from motor vehicle accidents associated with substance abuse—data very incomplete.

Process Objectives:

1. By 1987 each facility will have available outpatient, and residential treatment services for substance abuse.

2. By 1987 each facility will have a community awareness program regarding the problems associated with substance abuse and the treatment available. There should be at minimum a quarterly informational program. Special emphasis should be given to the school age child toward prevention.

X. Accident Prevention/Injury Control

Goal: *The number of injuries and fatalities from accidents will be reduced.*

Data Base: from OK-IHS-OEH

	1984	*National Goal*
1. Motor vehicle injuries	1163 (691 rate)	not established
2. Motor vehicle fatalities	42 (25 rate)	18/100,000
3. Motor vehicle fatalities for children under 5	1 (.5 rate)	5.5/100,000
4. Accident fatalities other than from motor vehicle accidents	29 (17.2 rate)	not established
5. Total fatalities from all accidents	71 (42.2 rate)	not established

Process Objectives:

1. By 1986, 90 percent of communities with a significant number of Indians will be served by a community injury control program.

2. All facilities should have a substance abuse program since a large number of accidents are associated with substance abuse (ref. IX).

3. By 1988 charts on 90 percent of all children under age two will contain evidence of accident prevention counseling (ref. IV, V).

4. By the end of 1986, infant seats will be available (see IV, 4).

5. All facilities should have safety as part of their employee orientation program and documented annual in-service.

6. By 1990, lost work days in Oklahoma IHS due to work-related injuries should be reduced.
   Data: 1985 lost work days in Oklahoma IHS = 16.6/100 rate (national goal = 55/100)

7. All facilities by the end of 1986 should have a functioning safety committee, with an injury surveillance system which gathers and analyzes data for an injury prevention program.

8. By 1987, each facility should have defined necessary and unnecessary diagnostic X-ray examinations and a quality assurance program should be in place to eliminate all unnecessary exams.

XI. Employee Health

Goal: *To prevent illness and to improve the health status of Oklahoma IHS employees. Lost work days due to illness and injury will be reduced.*

Data Base: 34.9 average sick hours per civil service employee in 1985; no accurate data available for commissioned officers.

Process Objectives:

1. By the end of 1986 all facilities will have an employee health program which includes preventive services (i.e., immunization, TB skin tests), a wellness component, employee assistance with substance abuse and mental health problems, stress reduction, emergency services, and environmental safety. There will also be a special emphasis program on women's health issues.

2. By 1987, 50 percent of all overweight employees will be attending a weight reduction program.

3. By 1987, 25 percent of all employees will particiate in an employee physical fitness program.

4. 50 percent of all IHS facilities will be smoke-free by 1986, and 100 percent by 1987.

5. By 1987, 50 percent of all IHS employees who are smokers will be offered a program to stop smoking and 50 percent will have completed a program by 1988. By 1990, 75 percent of those completing the program will remain smoke-free.

6. By 1987 all employees will have required rubella vaccine or have positive titers; all high-risk employees will have received hepatitis B vaccine; and by 1990, 60 percent of all employees have appropriately received diphtheria, tetanus, measles, mumps, influenza, and pneumococcal pneumonia vaccine (Ref. VII, 6).

7. Lost work days due to work-related injuries will be reduced (Ref. X, 6).

8. Commissioned officers will record all sick leave used to establish a data base, and this will be in place by the end of 1986.

XII. Stress and Violent Behavior

Goal: *To reduce the incidents of violent behavior, child abuse, suicide and homicide, and stress-related illnesses.*

Data Base:

- 1984 Oklahoma OSHD Statistics for Indians
  Suicide—11 cases (6.2 rate)
  Homicide—15 cases (8.9 rate)

- 1985 Oklahoma IHS discharges
  Suicide and self-inflicted injuries = 36 cases (21.4/100,000 rate)
  15 cases under age 20
  Homicide and injury purposely inflicted by other persons = 123
  (73.1/100,000 rate) 14 cases under age 20

- 1985 Oklahoma IHS outpatient visits
  Self-inflicted injuries = 49 (18 under age 20)
  Injuries purposely inflicted by other persons = 984 (291 under age 20)

Note: Data base on violent behavior, child abuse, and stress related illnesses
not available

Process Objectives:

1. By 1987, all facilities will develop a system for defining, identifying, and monitoring stress-related adverse advents.

2. By 1986 each facility will have full-time human services staff.

3. By 1987 all employee health programs will offer stress reduction seminars at least annually (Ref. XI, 1).

4. All facilities will have a functioning Child Abuse/Neglect Committee (Ref. V, 2).

5. By 1986 all facilities will have protocols for immediate care, and referral sources for:
   a. Child abuse/neglect
   b. Battered spouse
   c. Victims of sexual assault
   d. Emergency mental health services

Part 4

Medical Diagnosis Approach

Using Patient Outcomes to Evaluate Community Health Nursing

Frances Decker, Linda Stevens, Margaret Vancini, and Lorene Wedeking

Decker's article, published in 1979, provides a description of a successful statewide effort to develop indicators of the effectiveness of community health nursing through continued health care evaluation. It demonstrates the positive effect of the peer review process on nursing documentation and nurses' attitudes, by articulating the professional accountability that public health nurses at the local level assume for nursing care activities.

This three-year project carried out by the Community Nursing Section of the Minnesota Health Department provides excellent leadership in the development of local peer review committees using client outcome criteria in record audits. The project demonstrates that information about aggregate groups can be incorporated and shared with other agencies to promote the measurement of health status of communities or populations. Furthermore, the mechanism for record audit evalua-

tion reflects the way that the variability of situations and individuals affects nursing care. That is, the failure to achieve a health outcome is frequently justifiable and does not represent inappropriate nursing care.

The quality of health care today is of considerable interest to both recipients and providers. While both groups may have differing opinions as to what constitutes good health care, there seems to be agreement that such care is good if it positively alters the health status of the client who receives it. For this reason, much attention has been given by providers in the past decade to ways to measure health care. At first this was done by concentrating on evaluating the structure of the health care setting and, more recently, on evaluating the process and outcomes of the health care services given. The law creating professional Standards Review Organizations in 1972 gave impetus to this shift in emphasis and brought more order to the evaluation of health care in hospitals.[1] At the same time, attention also was being given to nonhospital services such as home health care, particularly by organized community health nursing services.[2]

That was the case with those of us in the community health nursing section of our state health department. In Minnesota, public health nursing services and home health care are available to clients in the state's 87 counties. Most of these services are provided by small, autonomous agencies, usually operating under local county auspices. Eight nurse consultants from our section provide consultation and technical assistance to staff public health nurses in these agencies through eight district offices. In 1974, the consultants reported that these nurses were expressing a need for help in developing an organized method of evaluating the quality of the care they were providing.

Specifically, the nurses were seeking a method that would help them identify (1) the kind of care provided by home health services, (2) ways it is being provided, and (3) the effectiveness of the care in creating positive change in the health status of the clients served. They also wanted a mechanism by which such data could be used to compare agencies, while respecting the confidentiality of each. Their last request was that the evaluation method be one that could be integrated into their ongoing agency review process and not be limited to a one-shot demonstration model.

TASKS TO BE COMPLETED

In order to meet this request, the community nursing section set up an advisory committee composed of staff from representative local nursing agencies, district public health nursing consultants, and other health professionals interested in the quality of care provided in the community. When the committee reviewed the literature concerning the quality assurance methodologies being used in the community health setting, they found relatively little to help them. In fact, as recently as 1977, Highriter, in summarizing research in community health nursing, noted the absence of indicators or tools for program evaluation.[3]

The advisory committee therefore concluded that to meet their objective several tasks would have to be completed. First, a feasible evaluation system had to be developed; next, a statewide education program for staff on how to use the system would have to be undertaken; then plans would have to be made for implementing and maintaining the system; and, finally, the system would have to be evaluated. At the recommendation of the advisory committee, the community nursing section undertook a three-year project, funded by the Northlands Regional Medical Programs, Inc., to undertake these tasks.

The first step in the project was to conduct a pilot study to determine what was to be evaluated. One obvious source of information about the health care provided was the clients' health care records. Nurses in six different agencies volunteered to participate in this phase of the project. However, rather than review every record, it was decided to concentrate on two of the most common services provided—care of the patient with a cerebral vascular accident and a postpartum woman.

In reviewing the past year's records for these patients, the group found 120 to 140 nursing process elements noted and 6 and 15 client health outcomes listed by each nurse for these patients. For example, nursing process included such activities as (for CVA) "taught patient transfer from bed to chair," "taught wife range of motion." For a postpartum patient, "explained recovery of the uterus and physiology of menses," "reviewed breast care." Outcomes were specific patient activities such as "patient moves from bed to chair, uses walker to bathroom," and "patient reports return of normal menses of 5-day duration, moderate to scant flow."

Unfortunately, in conducting the review for process and outcomes notes, the nurses found it took four-and-a-half hours to complete the task on each record. They concluded that it was too time consuming to review for both the process and outcome and decided to concentrate on patient outcomes only. Support for this decision can be found in ANA's *Guidelines for Review of Nursing Care at the Local Level,* in which the use of outcome criteria is credited with identifying the difference care makes for the client.[4]

DEVELOPING OUTCOME CRITERIA

In the second step of the project, 14 nurses participated in a three-stage seminar during which they developed outcome criteria for clients with presenting diagnoses of CVA and postpartum care. They then compared the criteria to 100 closed client health records from their agencies. Finally, on the basis of this comparison, they recommended corrective actions where needed. Several significant factors were identified as a result of this analysis.

First, the nurses found levels of agreement among themselves as to what the expected outcome criteria for a client's health status in these two categories—CVA and postpartum—would be. Second, the time involved in doing the evaluation was much shorter. Third, being able to demonstrate that in 90 of the 100 cases the client attained the expected health status was a positive experience for the nurses. Fourth, they realized that where a health outcome was not achieved, the cause often was outside of the nursing care the patient received. For instance, it might be because the patient was rehospitalized, moved, died, or so forth.

The nurses enthusiastically endorsed the use of outcome criteria, so the next step was to conduct a series of workshops statewide to teach nurses in the local community health agencies how to develop outcome criteria and to use these criteria in evaluating patient care.

A series of workshops consisting of three sessions were held in each of the eight health districts. A total of 251 nurses, representing 79 agencies, vlunteered to attend. During the workshops, 35 peer review committees were organized among the participants, and a registered record administrator was added to the project staff to assist these committees in retrieving data and preparing summary reports. Specifically, the peer review committees completed the following steps in the audit cycle: (1) developed criteria for designated groups of patients, such as CVAs; (2) compared closed records for patients within these groups to the criteria; (3) analyzed the records that did not meet these criteria; and (4) recommended corrective action.

At the completion of this process, 35 criteria sets covering six different health care conditions were completed. These conditions included adult diabetes mellitus, cancer of the lung, chronic arthritis, family planning, pediatric growth and development, and alcohol and drug abuse. Since many of these sets were duplicates of the same condition, they were condensed into six sets of what became known as "core criteria." The sets were eventually distributed to each participating agency.

During the evaluation process, 510 closed records were analyzed and the results compiled into a statewide summary. Approximately one half of the records surveyed met all of the outcome criteria. In the remaining half (213), four areas of deficiencies were found. The first and foremost was lack of documentation for the outcomes described in the criteria. In 128 instances, the reason was a lack of documentation in the charting; in 52 instances, it was a lack of clearly stated criteria; and, in 33 instances, nursing process or agency policy were detriments to the outcome of care.

A summary of these evaluation results was then sent to all participating agencies, where corrective actions could then be addressed by peer review committees or through district meetings. For example, the district nursing consultant could assist in organizing a district inservice meeting on problem-oriented recording or the discharge summary, rather than a single inservice program being held in each agency in her district.

AGGREGATE GROUPS

The need to focus on aggregate health care data in addition to individual client data in the community health setting has recently been addressed in an article by Williams.[5] By definition, community health nursing requires that information about nursing care to aggregate groups be incorporated into the measurement of health status of communities or populations. This led to starting a data bank in the community nursing section so that information about outcome criteria and audit findings could be shared with all the agencies. Such data were helpful, for instance, when two counties recently expanded services to newborns and parents. In addition to their own evaluation measures, the nurses involved in these services had access to core outcome criteria for newborn and postpartum care that were based on the outcomes expected by public health nurses throughout the state.

The next step in the project was to increase the criteria sets to cover more patient care conditions. For this reason, the 35 peer review committees reorganized themselves, with the assistance of the district consultants, into 32 ongoing committees. These committees then developed 120 sets of outcome criteria covering 33 different health care conditions (see Figs. 1 and 2 for samples) and conducted evaluations on over 600 client records using these criteria.

A permanent criteria and data collection and distribution system was set up at the community nursing section, enabling the peer review committees across the state to have access to a summary of health care evaluation data being generated in this process. Guidelines for forming and maintaining peer review committees conducting data analysis were developed and distributed to each agency.

Finally, as the system was put into operation at the local level, findings by individual agencies and peer review committees regarding the effects of nursing in the community health setting began to evolve. It was time to evaluate the total activities of the project.

GAINS ACHIEVED

There are a number of ways of looking at the accrued gains from this three-year project in addition to citing the yearly results which have been briefly described above. From the numerical standpoint, we can cite the following:

FIGURE 1
Sample Criteria Set

Topic:	Failure to thrive
Population:	Child aged 0-24 months with hisotry of delayed physical growth
Point in Time:	Discharge from community nursing program

1. Child develops a sense that environment can satisfy needs.
   a. Child vocalizes in age-appropriate manner as determined by developmental assessment tool.
   b. Child's range of affect expands to include smiling and ability to show displeasure (cry) during interaction with caregiver.
   c. Child demonstrates increased interest in people and environment as measured by number of contacts in 15-minute stimulation session.
   d. Child demonstrates positive eating experience by progressing from disinterest to enjoyment of both food and interaction with caregiver.

2. Child has progressive weight gain.
   a. Child's weight is at or above percentile of birthweight as determined by monthly weight checks.

3. Caregiver develops responses of nurturance of and support to child.
   a. Caregiver describes positive interaction with child.
   b. Caregiver lists at least two normal behaviors in four basic developmental areas (gross motor, fine motor, language, personal-social).
   c. Caregiver demonstrates increased nurturing behaviors.
   d. Caregiver demonstrates awareness of available support groups.
   e. Caregiver lists age-appropriate nutritional needs.

(1) over 400 nurses have become familiar with peer record review using outcome criteria; (2) across the state, 32 peer review committees are actively involved in health care evaluation; (3) all 39 sets of "core criteria" are now available statewide for committee use in health care evaluation; and (4) a total of 1,285 closed client records have been reviewed through 96 audit cycles. (An audit cycle begins with developing outcome criteria, and continues through comparing these criteria to records of patients with similar conditions, analyzing those records that do not meet the criteria, and making recommendations to correct the deficiencies found.) From a process standpoint, a statewide system of health care evaluation has been identified, taught, implemented, and evaluated within three years.

LONG-RANGE EFFECT

While acknowledging these results, we believe that the most important perspective on the outcomes of a project is whether the results have taken hold; that is, are there visible signs that the learning experience facilitated

FIGURE 2
Sample Criteria Set

Topic:	Congestive heart failure
Population:	Adult in own home
Point in Time:	Discharge from home health program

1. Cardiovascular status maintains stable pattern.
   a. Pulse rate between 60-90/min.
   b. Respiratory rate 15-24/min.—easy.
   c. Lung sounds clear.
   d. Body weight stable.
   e. Color of circumoral area and nailbeds pink.
   f. Breathes easily in supine position.
   g. Absence of edema in legs and feet.
   h. Can verbalize signs and symptoms that require consultation by doctor.
   i. Sees physician at prescribed intervals.

2. Working toward maximum activity and ADL independence.
   a. Plans rest periods.
   b. Has graduate program to maximize activity tolerance.
   c. Verbalizes environmental situations which influence CHF.
   d. Feeds, dresses, bathes, toilets self.
   e. Involves self in leisure activities within own tolerance.

3. Patient and/or significant other has knowledge of and eats prescribed diet.
   a. Prepares menus following prescribed diet.
   b. Lists restricted foods.
   c. Achieves and maintains optimum weight.
   d. Demonstrates ability to read food labels to identify those containing sodium.

4. Patient and/or significant other understands and follows medication regime.
   a. Takes meds at prescribed times.
   b. Demonstrates some standardized practice for taking meds at prescribed times.
   c. Distinguishes various medications.
   d. Explains actions of medications.
   e. Verbalizes signs and symptoms of toxicity of insufficient dose.

by the project made any changes in the attitudes and behaviors of the nurses who participated? One of the more observable changes noted by all those involved in some aspect of the project was an enthusiastic and positive attitude displayed by participants toward the health care evaluation process. The nurses quickly articulated that it was a clear system for taking professional responsibility for their nursing care activities. Like the nurses cited by Lohmann, they accepted the fact that the evaluation would illuminate their strengths as well as their weaknesses[6]. As one nurse commented on her evaluation sheet, "It was enlightening to find a way to show what nursing does that is positive instead of just showing what needs to be improved upon."

Participants also identified other potential uses of the data. For instance, it is being used (1) in agencies' annual reports to their funding sources, such as county commissioners; (2) to supply descriptive data to health planners in the state's Health Systems Agencies; (3) as one method for satisfying the evaluation requirements of a Minnesota Community Health Services subsidy; and (4) for planning district and state inservice programs on discharge planning and problem oriented recording, for example.

In individual agencies, the feedback from the health care evaluations has prompted a marked change in the discharge summaries of client records. Several agencies have implemented audit committees and record committees that have designed a series of flow sheets to augment the outcome criteria sets. Strikingly, almost every agency has begun considering additional methodologies for appraising the nursing process, especially in instances where the outcome evaluations have indicated a need for assessment of the process.

For example, if it is determined during a peer review evaluation that a diabetic client has not learned to administer his insulin, this finding alerts the nurses to go back and inspect the process of care as it was documented in order to identify and correct the missing portion in the care process. At times it may be a problem with recording; at other times it may mean a need for more or better teaching.

Initially, the nurses had been concerned that the variability in the situations and individuals they encounter would interfere with developing statements about the outcomes of health care for specific patients. After completing several evaluations, they were surprised to find that the new mechanism reflects how the variability of situations and individuals affects nursing care. They had thought they would be held accountable for the impossible task of controlling all such variables.

An illustration of this point can be seen in the summary of justified variations—that is, the determination by the peer review committee that the failure to achieve a health outcome does *not* represent inappropriate nursing care. During the final project year, 130 such variables were found. The largest source of justified variation (32 percent) was the presence of secondary diagnoses which interfered in some way with achievement of health outcomes designated for a group of persons having the same primary diagnosis. Other important sources of justified variation were the refusal of services by the client (15 percent) and the transfer of the client to an institution or different geographic area before nursing goals were achieved (15 percent). The nurses concluded that documenting and understanding the effect of such variables was the appropriate role for community health nursing at the present time, not the attempt to control the variables.

Another concern voiced by many was that the scope of the project as a statewide endeavor was overambitious and might be prone to system breakdown. However, the support mechanism inherent in coordinating the local peer review committees' activities through the consulting staff of the community nursing section was rated as necessary by the nurses. They cited this method as a means of providing continuity in the evaluation activities during staff turnover and agency program changes. Their need for support resulted in the integration of the project staff positions into the community nursing section on a permanent basis.

Involving local nurses on a statewide basis is consistent with the philosophy of the community nursing section. The value of this has been reinforced by Goran, who states, "We have come to recognize that effective quality assurance cannot be mandated from on high. . . The federal government can provide the framework and tools to facilitate the efforts, but the real work must be done at the local level."[7]

PROFESSIONAL RESPONSIBILITY

At the same time, we believe community health nursing shares in the responsibility of the entire profession to develop quality assurance methods. Phaneuf sees that community health nursing has a special responsibility because current efforts are largely hospital and medically oriented. Anticipating that quality assurance activities will some day be mandatory for home health care, she writes, "Unless wise leadership effectively intervenes, patterns now being met will be followed beyond inpatient hospital walks. . ."[8]

Although we recognize that assessing the quality of community health nursing care by using outcome criteria for peer record review is not the only possible method of evaluation, it has been beneficial for nursing agencies in our state. One unexpected result has been the growing awareness on the part of both staff and project participants that the outcome of implementing a system of health care evaluation has in fact become a beginning. The agencies are now looking at how to improve nursing in other aspects of quality assurance such as the assessment process, discharge planning, problem-oriented recording, and multidisciplinary auditing. Most important, there now exists a clear demonstration of the need to devlop indicators of the effectiveness of community health nursing through continued health care evaluation. All of these beginnings will in turn bring the benefits of health care evaluation even closer to the logical recipient—the client.

ABOUT THE AUTHORS

At the time of writing, Frances Decker, MPH, RN, was Chief, Linda Stevens, BA, was Registered Record Administrator, and Lorene Wedeking, MS, RN, was Coordinator of Quality Assurance Activities, Community Nursing Section, Office of Community Health Services, Minnesota Department of Health, Minneapolis. Margaret Vancini, MS, RN, was Assistant Professor, School of Nursing, University of Wisconsin—

Au Claire, and was formerly coordinator of the peer review project, Community Health Nursing Section, Minnesota Department of Health.

REFERENCES

1. M. J. Goran, "The Future of Quality Assurance in Health Care: Next Steps from the Perspective of the Federal Government," *Bulletin of the New York Academy of Medicine,* 52 (January 1976), 177–184.

2. M. C. Phaneuf, *The Nursing Audit: Self-Regulation in Nursing Practice* (New York: Appleton-Century-Crofts, 1976).

3. M. E. Highriter, "The Status of Community Health Nursing Research," *Nursing Research,* 26 (May-June 1977), 183–192.

4. *Guidelines for Review of Nursing Care at the Local Level* (Kansas City, MO: American Nurses' Association, 1976).

5. C. A. Williams, "Community Health Nursing—What is It?" *Nursing Outlook,* 25 (April 1977), 250–254.

6. Grace Lohmann, "A Statewide System of Record Audit," *Nursing Outlook,* 25 (May 1977), 330–332.

7. Goran, "The Future of Quality Assurance in Health Care."

8. Phaneuf, *The Nursing Audit.*

Outcome Criteria: Public Health Nursing and Home Care Services

Minnesota Department of Health

The outcome criteria presented here, developed by the Public Health Nursing Section of the Minnesota Department of Health in Minneapolis, are examples of criteria based on the framework presented in the preceding article. These outcome criteria provide a working reference for a variety of specific medical diagnoses and patient populations.

TOPIC: GERIATRIC MAINTENANCE

Population: 65 + years

1. Client achieves ADLs with or without assistance.

   Client is able to do the following within limits of present condition with or without assistance.

Reprinted with permission from *Outcome Criteria: Public Health Nursing Services and Home Health Care Services* (Minneapolis: Public Health Nursing Section, Community Health Services Division, Minnesota Department of Health, revised October 1986).

1a. Eats

1b. Bathes

1c. Dresses

1d. Ambulates

1e. Maintains household

2. Client copes with aging and/or disease process.

2a. Client verbalizes feelings.

2b. Client interacts with significant others.

3. Client and/or family have adquate medical supervision.

3a. Client contacts doctor periodically, i.e., every three months.

4. Client maintains adequate physical status.

4a. Client eats well-balanced diet.

4b. Client maintains satisfactory body weight according to physician/nurse.

4c. Client indicates participation in physical activity.

5. Client receives adequate financial support.

5a. Client demonstrates financial status is adequate for needs.

5b. Client demonstrates awareness of resources available if help is necessary.

Note: See also criteria on Nutrition of Aged

TOPIC: OPEN WOUND REQUIRING DRESSING CHANGE

Population: Adult

1. Client and/or significant other understands healing process and its effects.

1a. Client and/or significant other describes cause of wound.

1b. Client and/or significant other describes healing process.

1c. Client and/or significant other describes signs of complications of healing.

1d. Client and/or significant other relates healing process to own wound and own prognosis of healing.

2. Client and/or significant other understands management of healing process.

2a.   Client and/or significant other lists wound-related medications used and side effects of each medication.

2b.   Client and/or significant other describes treatment of wound including dressing change utilizing principles of asepsis.

2c.   Client and/or significant other describes plan for use in case of complications of wound healing.

2d.   Client and/or significant other verbalizes the significance of appropriate diet for wound healing.

2e.   Client and/or significant other describes adjustments in activities to promote healing.

3.   Client and/or significant other implements a management program, independently as able.

3a.   Client and/or significant other complies with medication regime.

3b.   Client and/or significant other carries out treatment of wound and dressing changes using principles of asepsis.

3c.   Client increases intake of protein and vitamin C foods and increases intake of fluids from pre-wound status to promote healing.

3d.   Client adjusts activities to promote healing.

4.   Client accepts necessary life style adjustments.

4a.   Client verbalizes positive/negative feelings about changed body image, drainage, pain, odor, and activity limitations imposed by wound.

4b.   Client seeks assistance, if needed.

4c.   Client sees physician for follow-up wound care, as needed.

5.   Client's wound is healing and free of infection and pain.

5a.   The wound has an absence of redness, discharge, swelling, or foul odor.

5b.   Client states pain and tenderness in wound is decreased.

5c.   Depth of diameter of wound is decreased.

TOPIC: TERMINALLY ILL PATIENT; TERMINALLY ILL CANCER PATIENT

Population: Adult

1.   Client achieves or maintains optimal comfort level.

1a. Client or significant other utilizes comfort measures to relieve pain (position changes, air mattress, sheepskin, etc.).

1b. Client takes prescribed medication as required.

1c. Client or significant other explains purpose, effects, and side effects of medications.

1d. Client communicates that pain is controlled within tolerable limits.

2. Client maintains optimum physical status.

2a. Client or significant other provides or adapts personal care measures.

2b. Client ingests food and fluids.

2c. Client controls nausea and vomiting (if applicable).

2d. Client utilizes special equipment and supplies as needed (wheelchair, hospital bed, disposable pads, etc.).

3. Client copes with illness and dying.

3a. Client demonstrates awareness of and preparation for physical changes caused by illness.

3b. Client or significant other discusses available community resources.

3c. Client is involved in decisions about care (use of medications, place of death, life support measures, etc.)

3d. Client plans and talks about how family will manage after death.

3e. Client communicates feelings of a part or all of the grieving process to significant others (denial, anger, bargaining, depression, acceptance).

4. Family members and significant others cope with client's illness and approaching death.

4a. Family and significant others plan and talk with client about how family will manage after death.

4b. Family and significant others communicate feelings of a part or all of the grieving process.

Quality Assurance in a Home Health Agency

Joan Buddi

Accountability for the quality of care provided by community health agencies is receiving increased scrutiny. The following piece presents the viewpoint of a home health agency nurse administrator. Buddi describes how statewide standards for home health care were established in Florida. The article defines the responsibility for determining quality of care from the perspective of a corporate entity. The outcome audit developed in Florida is premised upon a sound philosophy, and Buddi describes several steps in determining audit methodology.

INTRODUCTION

Administrative accountability of community health providers far exceeds that required in any other sector of society or business. The reasons for this are many. Foremost among them is modern technology which has created a myriad of sophisticated diagnostic tools, complicated treatments and complex medications. As consumers of health care become more knowledgeable

Reprinted from *Community Health Nursing: Education and Practice*, copyright © 1980, National League for Nursing, New York, pp. 61-71.

of their health needs, their perspectives on health care providers are shifting from that of a trusting complacency to an insistence on accountability. Unfortunately, the issue of accountability is most frequently raised in situations which bring into question the safe provision of quality care. Only when deficiencies are noted is accountability examined. Health care providers have been inconsistent in responding to consumer demand for accountability. Some have declined to consider new techniques to facilitate accountability, relying instead on existing professional codes of ethics and licensing requirements.

Coinciding with the advances of medical science, the labor movement has demanded and won health care provisions for employees, resulting in a variety of health care programs established by state and federal governments. This increase in third-party payers, the involvement of billions of federal dollars, and a laxity by health professionals in establishing accountability controls have led to a multitude of complex regulations. These regulations have been established with the objective of ensuring that the care provided is appropriate and cost-effective; however, it is questionable whether these objectives have been met.

In the past, health institutions have been subject to intense scrutiny by regulatory boards, and precise procedures have been established to determine and ensure that obligations to consumers, third-party payers, and the federal government are met. The focus is now shifting to community health care.

PERSONAL EXPERIENCE

As a professional nurse and administrator of a home health agency, I tend to agree with Webster's definitions of the terms "responsible" and "accountable," which in essence is "being liable to be called upon or able to answer for one's conduct and obligations." In my role as administrator, I have categorized my obligations to those to whom I am accountable. The consumer has a right to expect the highest quality of care available within the constraints of applicable rules and regulations. The community has a right to expect the agency to contribute to the welfare of that society by performing within the bounds of the agency's purpose. The employees, as professionals, can expect the agency to provide an atmosphere conducive to achieving quality patient care as well as job satisfaction. Other health care providers and facilities have the right to know how a particular agency interrelates and interacts with the purposes of other institutions; to know the agency's functions, limitations, and philosophy for health care. The local, state, and federal agencies and fiscal intermediaries, of course, expect the proper execution of their respective requirements.

In addition to establishing these categories, I have attempted to specify three areas of accountability—program accountability, fiscal accountability and procedural accountability. The three are interrelated and it would be folly to place a greater emphasis on any one more than another. Both traditional and modern management techniques are used to aid in meeting the demands for accountability in these categories and to achieve a balance of flexibility and stability.

However, there are areas of ambiguity. To be accountable for quality patient care, quality patient care must first be adequately defined. Such definition is not a task to be undertaken by an administrator only. Even nurses would have difficulty formulating the definition, setting standards, or attempting to evaluate professional action.

DETERMINING QUALITY CARE

Recently, the Florida Association of Home Health Agencies, Inc., established a Quality Assurance Committee. The committee was comprised of home health agency nurses representing the entire state, and its purpose was to establish statewide standards for home health care in Florida. Much research was done before the committee determined which route to pursue in the development of standards and a method of assuring quality patient care. The existing literature was reviewed and three types of audit were clearly defined.

The first was the structure audit, which applies to the setting in which care is given. It focuses on physical facilities, equipment, the personnel providing the care, and the institution's organization. Rules and policies governing the professional work and medical records are reviewed. The structure audit is based on the proposition that given reasonable standards of facilities and organization, good health care is likely to prevail, and excellence in structure results in excellence of care. As promising as this sounds, limited research is available to confirm this assumption.

The process audit is the second type. In this approach, the auditor observes what happens and the order in which certain events occur. Process audit information is collected either by direct observation or record review. It determines if the professional subject to the audit has performed his/her duties properly and is thus a very "task oriented" type of audit. The problem encountered is the lack of defined standards. Professional judgments on the process of care are difficult to make because of conflicting views about the process itself and the variety of standards used.

The third type of audit is the most recently developed. The outcome audit reviews the status of the patient after care is provided. It is performed retrospectively and seeks to determine how the care provided has affected the patient. The difficulty with outcome audit is in defining "outcome."

The committee, in its effort to formulate standards of home health care, reviewed existing rules, regulations and laws in the state. The first to be reviewed was Florida's Nurse Practice Act, signed into law by Governor Reuben Askew in 1975. The act states its purpose and makes reference to accountability:

> . . . in order to safeguard the life, health and welfare of the people in this state and to protect them from unauthorized, unqualified and improper application of services by individuals engaging in the practice of nursing.
>
> The professional nurse and the practice nurse shall be responsible and accountable for making decisions that are based upon the individual's educational preparation and experiences in nursing.''

The Florida Nurse Practice Act set only minimum requirements for education and licensure. It did, however, define the responsibilities of the Board of Nursing and charged the board to enforce the provisions of the law.

FURTHER RESEARCH

The State of Florida has a licensing law for home health agencies. Known as Rules of the Department of Health & Rehabilitative Services (Division of Health) Minimum Standards for Home Health Agencies, the standards contained in the law serve as the basis for structural and process-type audits. However, the standards cannot validly be used to assess the quality of patient care provided; neither can those standards contained in Conditions of Participation in the Medicare Program. The American Nurses' Association's *Standards of Nursing Practice* were also reviewed, but the committee determined that these too were not specific enough for application to home health care. Finally, the committee decided that a diagnosis/outcome type of audit would provide the best mechanism for defining desired levels of patient care. Nineteen diagnosis/outcome criteria, protocol for the audit and the forms with which to perform the audit were developed.

THE OUTCOME AUDIT

The primary goal in developing a patient care audit system was to provide a standard by which each agency could evaluate the care rendered by the professionals within the agency. A home care philosophy was formulated with the premise that patients have certain, basic rights and that health care professionals are responsible and accountable for setting standards of care, rendering the care, and evaluating the care. That patient care depends upon a multifaceted program of planning, educating, and communicating, done by representatives of each distinct health care profession, is another basic tenet of home health care's philosophy.

The outcome audit, as peer review, is an organized and systematic method that evaluates the care patients receive and the abilities of professionals who provide care. It can determine if and how professional intervention affects the health status of the patient.

The committee established objectives for each audit:

- To determine the actual performance as related to the developed outcome criteria.
- To identify strengths and deficiencies in patient care documentation.
- To determine if developed criteria are realistic.
- To determine and delegate appropriate corrective action and provide follow-up evaluation to ensure that action has been taken.
- To report results to the executive committee, chief executive officer, and/or governing body of the agency.

There are several steps in audit methodology. The first is to establish outcome criteria that accurately measure the patient care provided by the nursing staff. Outcome is considered an alteration in the health status of the consumer. It is the end result of activities (process) performed by the professional and not the activities themselves. Sound criteria must be measurable, realistic, achievable, clinically sound, predetermined, positive, objective, understandable, and have identifiable commonalities. The outcome criteria that the committee developed were based on medical diagnosis or disease entities.

As the committee criteria were being developed, it was found helpful to organize criteria for certain patient populations into subsets or headings, based on categories of concern. Although not absolutely necessary, criteria subsets are useful in organizing the development of criteria and also help to assure that all aspects of patient care are provided for in the listing of outcome criteria. (E.g., the criteria subsets were labeled physical [which includes disease process and state of comfort], safety, psychosocial, and educational.) When criteria are listed under the heading to which they pertain, the process is more organized and easier to work within.

OTHER NEEDS

Patient populations must be specific and well defined; variables or characteristics desired must be indicated. In conducting an audit, variables must be selected to reduce the population being studied and make the group more homogenous and tractable. The number of variables must be large enough to identify a patient population with similar characteristics, yet small enough so that enough patients can be found that fit the characteristics. Data regarding the variables should be available and retrievable.

Among the criteria should be the desired percentage of conformance. The recommended standard to be used is 100 percent. If this standard is set, all cases not meeting this level must be examined and a reason determined for the lack of achievement. In order to justify setting 100 percent as the desired conformance percentage, one must clinically identify justifiable exceptions.

The next step in outcome audit methodology is measurement. The measurement of actual practice against the established criteria will produce reliable data. A defined objective method for measurement and inclusion of all, or a representative sample, of patients (random sampling of 10-20 records with same diagnosis) will also help render reliable data. The results of measurement must then be analyzed by peers. Analysis requires identification of conformance to and variations from the criteria; explicit justification for all variations that are clinically acceptable; identification of deficiencies in the provision of patient care, and attribution of the deficiencies to their sources.

This leads, naturally, to the next step—action. Action must be taken to overcome the deficiencies identified, being specific to the deficiencies and effective in accomplishing change. Action taken should be non-punitive, such as counseling; inservice education; staffing; patient education; policies and procedures; or new forms for medical records. These are all things that can be done in a positive way to correct the identified deficiencies.

After appropriate action has been taken, the next step is reevaluation. Follow-up must be immediate if life threatening, and documented to show improvement in patient care. All action taken must be reevaluated to determine whether it was effective. Individual professional counseling may be given, but if the desired change is not effected, then a group inservice education program may have to be initiated.

The audit results must be reported following reevaluation. This means that general findings and specific recommendations are accurately stated and recorded. This report should be acknowledged by the professional advisory board, the governing board, the chief executive officer, and the director of nursing staff. The report being retained as a permanent administrative record allows for accountability.

PURPOSE OF THE AUDIT

The objective of outcome audit, as a peer review, is neither to punish or to accumulate an impressive amount of papers and documents. It is to determine weaknesses and strengths; give direction for appropriate educational programs; and through education and reeducation, enhance the strengths and reduce the weaknesses. This is how quality of patient care will be improved and how professionals can demonstrate their ability to handle responsibility and be accountable for the quality of care.

The outcome audit program is one of evaluation devised to promote excellence of service. This excellence is possible through systematic, ongoing evaluation and continuous action for improvement. It is designed to guarantee to the consumer, family, and community an achievable and realistic level of health care. It acknowledges and accepts the agency's responsibility to predict outcome of care, to measure the results of services and to initiate corrective action. However, a complete quality assurance program will also include structure audits and process audits.

An important reason for establishing an outcome audit program is to define standards of care that can be communicated to consumers. The effect of care on the consumer can be identified and standards of care established based upon the expected health status of patients at time of discharge. Objectives formulated can be applied to each and every audit performed, regardless of geography.

THE LIMITATIONS OF AUDIT

As standards were developed for the audit, it became apparent that an important aspect of understanding an audit procedure is to recognize what an audit is and what it is not. An audit is a systematic method of measuring the quality of patient care as it is reflected in the patient's medical record. It is a vehicle to meet the increasing demands for accountability that have been placed upon the entire health care delivery system; an instrument to measure and evaluate; and a technique of using clinical observations of a group of similar patients to detect patterns of care.

An audit should not be an agency's total quality assurance program. Other evaluation activities might include a checklist of the mechanics of charting, patient questionnaires, performance assessment, and an ongoing monitoring of the processes of care. Audit is not a replacement for effective supervision or managerial skills, nor is it a utilization review (which examines individual charts and questions the justification of services).

There are several benefits to be gained from initiating the outcome audit. Perhaps the most important is the upgrading of patient care by improving staff practices. Once outcome criteria are established, a standard is set which staff members strive to attain, thus improving patient care.

Any deficiencies in written policies or procedures are revealed by the audit. Because the audit reviews outcomes of care and measures the outcomes to the standard, existing deficiencies will become apparent. If a staff member follows agency policy and procedure and still demonstrates a deficiency, perhaps the policy and/or procedure require change rather than the staff member.

Coordination of the entire health care team is another benefit. Communication with and utilization of other community services is enhanced. Once again, when a specific desired outcome is determined, the patient's needs are made known, as well as needs anticipated after discharge. More utilization of community resources and increased communication result.

The audit also provides standards for more pertinent documentation of patient care. This type of quality assurance program facilitates reimbursement, role identification, and improved care. The outcome criteria is stated in patient behavioral terms, and therefore requires that specific items be referenced in documentation. The chart then describes a patient's status with more specificity and accuracy.

When specific strengths and weaknesses are identified, areas of educational need are indicated. The programs developed will improve patient care by improving professional staff competence. When deficiencies are identified, their reason must be ascertained. If not for faulty education, on occasion, the agency's internal quality assurance committee may be able to demonstrate, with specific documentation, that additional personnel are needed.

Researchable aspects of patient care may also be found through the outcome audit. For example, agency internal committees will be able to evaluate, on a process audit, the effectiveness of certain supplies or patient teaching tools.

All these benefits of the outcome audit are in addition to its purpose—to provide a method of accountability to governing bodies and the consuming public.

IMPLEMENTING AUDITS

The outcome criteria for audit have now been established for skilled nursing. Most nursing staff are receptive to this type of program and use the established criteria as a basis for preparation of patient care plans. Since the program is still young, long-term benefits can only be anticipated. Perhaps the biggest problem in implementation of the program is a sense of discouragement felt by some staff after reviewing actual performance results. They often fall short of the ideal. Fortunately, such discouragement is usually overcome as staff performance improves.

Nursing staff are now eagerly awaiting criteria being developed by physical therapists and speech therapists. The physical therapists are developing criteria for 18 diagnoses and the speech therapists have already developed criteria for three diagnoses. The eventual goal is for each agency in the state of Florida to perform a multidisciplinary patient care outcome audit, all using the same standards.

An awareness of the need for quality maintenance in home health agencies and an understanding of outcome audit methodology are important prerequisites to an effective patient care audit. However, there is another element vital to the actual implementation of an auditing system. To be successful, audits must have the active support of the agency governing body and a majority of its administrators and practitioners.

Retrospective chart audit is another systematic method by which health professionals and institutions can review and improve their performance, and thereby improve patient care. Practitioners follow set criteria, analyze variations and decide upon corrective action for deficiencies. But despite the fact that it is the professionals under review who make the system work, the ultimate legal responsibility for ensuring this activity lies with the agency's governing authority. The reason for this is readily apparent. Even though health care professionals, such as nurses and physical therapists, have a direct stake in quality maintenance through their professional activities and are vulnerable to malpractice suits for substandard care, *it is the agency, as a corporate entity, that is fundamentally responsible for the overall successful functioning of the organization.*

Basic to the very concept of corporate responsibility is the governing body's moral obligation to those it serves. In a home health agency setting, the governing authority has the obligation to assure that the resources it controls are utilized for the advantage and well-being of those seeking the organization's assistance. This obligation means that the agency's governing body, as the legal personification of the corporate entity, bears the ultimate responsibility for quality maintenance. In terms of patient care audit, therefore, the governing body's role is to assure that audits are properly conducted, that the results are documented and reviewed at all appropriate levels, and that the correct action is taken. This is a continuing responsibility that directors should assume as part of their leadership duties, even though they may not be health care professionals.

In order for the governing body to effectively exercise responsibility for ensuring effective audit implementation, it must devote adequate time to reviewing each audit completed by practitioners. Although the ultimate responsibility is the governing body's, monitoring quality of care and cost review activities within the home health agency, including audit and utilization review, may sometimes be delegated. Recommended actions of the audit committee should be approved by the director of nursing service or a designated representative, who may be a member of the audit committee. The audit committee must keep itself informed of all corrective action taken, thus facilitating evaluation of the appropriateness of its recommendations. A summary of audit activities should then be reported to the governing board through the chief executive officer.

CONCLUSION

No longer is quality assurance a purely professional need. Quality assurance is a *public* need, required for the defense of the entire health care system by enhancing its credibility. Programs such as the audit outcome are becoming mandatory because consumers of health care are demanding that health care providers be accountable for the services they provide. Society grants to health professionals considerable authority over functions vital to the commonweal and allows much autonomy in the control of their own affairs. In return, the health professional is expected to act responsibly, always mindful of its public trust and accountable for its own practices. Self-regulation and self-discipline are recognized as hallmarks of professionalism, and home health agencies should not endanger their survival or independence by ignoring their responsibilities.

ABOUT THE AUTHOR

Joan Buddi, MS, RN, is Administrator, Home Health Agency of North Broward, Tamarac, Florida.

Quality Assurance Program

Florida Association of Home Health Agencies

*The directions for the Florida outcome audit described in the preceeding
article by Buddi are reprinted here in full to provide an indepth look
at implementation of written outcome criteria by medical diagnosis.
The Florida Association of Home Health Agencies describes a step-by-
step process to implement the outcome audit procedure, and provides
a method of accountability for the community health agency governing
body and to the public. Recommended forms for use in the outcome
audit process are provided. Finally, we have included one example of
skilled nursing outcome criteria—that for care of an open wound.*

INTRODUCTION

Consumers of health care, providers of health care, and payers of health
care are expressing concerns regarding the quality of care rendered. This increase of awareness by the public is demonstrated by the consumers exercising

the rights to question the providers of health care about the extent, type, cost and alternatives in the care provided. The health care professionals have recognized the increasing degree of accountability for which they are held responsible, and the payers of health care want to know what has been purchased and if the care provided has been appropriate for the stated diagnosis or condition. Consequently, there is no longer a choice, but a mandate to implement a program for the determination of "quality" in health care, more specifically, home health care.

Quality is defined as a degree of excellence, while the definition of assurance is the act or action of pledging or guaranteeing. Therefore to establish a quality assurance program is to devise an audit method "to pledge a degree of excellence."

Several different audit methodologies have been devised in attempts to verify the quality of health care rendered. The structure audit focuses on the framework of the organization in which care is given, rules and policies governing the professiosnal work and medical records. It is based on the assumption that given reasonable standards of facilities and organization, good health care may be expected to be rendered.

The process audit is the second type of audit, wherein the auditor examines an event as it occurs and the order in which it occurs. The process audit is very task oriented and determines if the health care provider has performed assigned duties "appropriately." This, then presents the concern of defining standards, as professional judgments of the "process of care" are often different.

The third type of audit is called outcome or retrospective audit; which reviews the status of the patient at the time of discharge, from service, in relationship to the effect of the care rendered prior to discharge. It seeks to determine what effect did the care given have in changing the health status of the patient. The difficulty with the outcome audit is defining the desired "outcome."

The Quality Assurance Committee decided that the outcome type of audit would be the most beneficial for the recipients of home health care in the state of Florida. The task then became one of developing a method to do an outcome audit in a home health agency, develop appropriate forms, and most importantly write the desired patient outcome status according to medical diagnosis. The medical diagnosis was utilized to simplify medical record material and to facilitate joint services (skilled nursing, physical therapy and speech pathology) audit. The medical diagnosis would be a common denominator and would be retrievable in any home health agency.

OUTCOME AUDIT

Written outcome criteria by medical diagnosis also meant determining specific physical, safety, psychosocial, and educational levels desired for each patient at the time of discharge. To compare how that patient actually was at time of discharge against the specific written criteria required the establishment of a standard of 100 percent conformance to the criteria. Should the standard of 100 percent conformance not be met, the deficiencies would exist which would require corrective action. With this flow of activities, the committee established objectives for each audit which would be performed in any given agency:

- To determine the actual performance related to developed outcome criteria for the stated diagnosis.

- To identify strengths and deficiencies in patient care documentation, attesting to quality of care.

- To determine if developed criteria are realistic.

- To determine and delegate appropriate corrective action and provide follow-up evaluation to insure that action has been taken.

- To report to executive committee and/or governing body of the agency and chief executive officer.

Certain advantages can be expected as a result of the implementation of an outcome audit method for quality assurance. These benefits might include, but are not limited to:

- Improving patient care by improving staff practices. The outcome criteria describes the desired state for a patient at the time of discharge, thus the staff will strive for this state.

- Demonstrating deficiencies of written policies and/or procedures.

- Encouraging more coordination of the health care team.

- Improving communication with and utilization of other community services.

- Providing standards for more pertinent documentation of patient care rendered, which will facilitate:
  1. Role identification
  2. Improved care
  3. Reimbursement

- Providing direction for educational programs which will be geared to improving quality and professional competence.

- Identifying areas where additional personnel are needed.

- Identifying specific aspects of patient care for research by providing factual data to demonstrate the level of care rendered.

- Providing a method of accountability for the governing body and to the public.

METHODOLOGY: SIX BASIC STEPS OF OUTCOME AUDIT

The first step in the establishment of an outcome audit is to *develop outcome criteria*. Outcome is an alteration in the health status of the patient. It is the end result of activities (process) performed by the professionals and not the activities in and of themselves. To develop outcome criteria there are specific considerations. The criteria must be measureable, realistic, achievable, clincially sound, predetermined, positive in nature, objective, use clear concise terms, and have identifiable commonalities.

In actual performance of the audit procedure, patient populations must be specific and well defined. Each individual agency who utilizes this procedure must predetermine these patient populations or "variables." The variables should be selected to reduce the population being studied to make the group more homogenous. Examples of variables are: age, sex, race, health history, or geographic boundries.

The number of variables should be large enough to identify a patient population with similar characteristics, yet small enough for trend identification. Variables must be selected for which data is available and retrievable.

In order to complete the criterion, the desired percentage of conformance must be included. The recommended standard is 100 percent; by setting this standard, all cases not meeting this must be examined and reviewed to determine a reason for the lack of achievement. To realistically substantiate setting 100 percent as the desired conformance percentage, clinically justifiable exceptions must be identified.

Measurement of actual practice against the predetermined criteria is the second step of the outcome audit methodology. Measurement requires comparing actual practice to the criteria to produce reliable data.

The third step is *analysis*, the results of measurement by peers. Analysis requires identification of conformance to and of variations from the criteria, explicit justifications for all variations that are clinically acceptable, and perhaps most importantly, identification of deficiencies in the provision of patient care and attribution of these deficiencies by their source.

Action is the fourth step of the audit procedure. Action must be taken to overcome the deficiencies identified. It must be specific to the deficiencies identified and effective in accomplishing change. Action, positive in nature, should be non-punitive such as counseling, inservice education, and patient education.

Appropriate action is followed by the fifth step, *reevaluation* in order to determine if the action taken has been effective in correcting the identified deficiencies.

The final and sixth step is to *report* the audit results. General findings of the audit and specific recommendations are accurately stated and recorded. It should be acknowledged by the executive committee of the agency, chief executive officer, and director of nursing service. The report should be retained as a permanent administrative record.

Figure 1 displays the actions of the Florida Association of Home Health Agencies, Inc., Quality Assurance Committee and the outcome audit methodology.

IMPLEMENTATION OF THE OUTCOME AUDIT PROCEDURE IN AN INDIVIDUAL HOME HEALTH AGENCY

An awareness of the need for quality maintenance in the home health agency, along with an understanding of outcome audit methodology are important prerequisites to an effective patient care audit, but they lack an element vital to the actual implementation of a functioning audit system. To be successful, implementation must have the active and majority support of the agency's practitioners, its administration, and its governing body.

FIGURE 1
The Audit Process

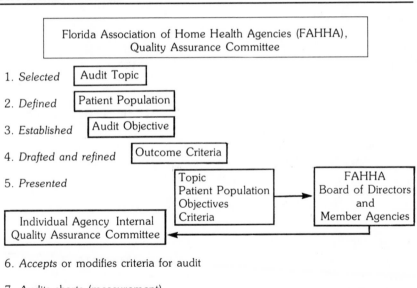

6. *Accepts* or modifies criteria for audit

7. *Audits* charts (measurement)

8. *Analyzes* variations

9. Takes corrective *action*

10. *Reevaluates*

11. *Reports* to administration

monitors implementation and *documents* changes in policy/practice/outcomes

Retrospective chart audit is a systematic method by which health professionals and institutions can review and improve their performance, and thereby improve patient care. Practitioners have set criteria, analyzed variations, and decided upon corrective action for deficiencies. But despite the fact that it is the professionals under review who make the system work, the ultimate legal responsibility for ensuring this activity lies with the agency's governing authority. The reason for this is readily apparent. Even though health care professionals such as nurses and physical therapists have a direct stake in quality maintenance through their professional activities and are vulnerable to malpractice suits for substandard care, it is the agency as a corporate entity that is fundamentally responsible for the overall successful functioning of the organization. Basic to the very concept of corporate responsibility is the governing body's moral obligation to those in whose behalf it serves. In a home health agency setting, the governing authority has the obligation to assure that the resources it controls are utilized to the advantage and for the well-being of those seeking the assistance the organization offers. This obligation means that the agency's governing body, as the legal personification of the corporate entity, bears the ultimate responsibility for quality maintenance.

In terms of patient care audit, therefore, the governing body's role is to assure that audits are done, that the results are documented and reviewed at all appropriate levels, and that appropriate action is taken. This is a continuing responsibility, and it is one that directors must assume, even though they may not be health care professionals.

In order for the governing body to exercise its ultimate responsibility for ensuring effective audit implementations, it must spend adequate time reviewing each audit as it is completed by the practitioners.

An agency internal Quality Assurance Committee should be established and have specific duties and obligations defined. The committee should be comprised of field personnel and at least one administrative person. The duties might include, but not be limited to: review of FAHHA's outcome criteria for revision and/or adaption, (or new outcome criteria may be written). It is suggested that a schedule for audit topics be prepared in the early phase of the committee and that the audit topics which are selected be by the medical diagnoses which are more commonly admitted to the agency.

When the committee has performed an audit and identified deficiencies, the corrective action must be specific. For example a person must be named to whom a task has been delegated; and a specific time/date set for completion of the action/task. Documentation must be kept of the action, including the person to whom the task was delegated and time of completion. The person completing the task should acknowledge the task completion by signing the appropriate committee form. This is how the outcome audit procedure provides a method of accountability for the governing body and to the public.

FURTHER CONSIDERATIONS

Peer review of the individual is a difficult process, and more often than not, is carried out on an informal rather than a formal basis. It operates as a laissez-faire system and frequently professionals are unwilling to pass any type of judgment on one another. To be accountable and responsible to our patients means to protect the patient from incompetent practitioners and to assume responsibility for improving the practice of health care professionals. Caution must be exercised to adopt a method of peer review which demonstrates a full commitment to the patient's well being, and acceptance of accountability for ourselves as individuals with responsibility for and to our respective professions.

In home health care, we experience a unique relationship with our patients in that we play many roles: scientific artists, teachers and counselors—scientific artists in the skills that each of us possess and perform each time we are in the home; teachers that bring knowledge to a patient and family so that they are able to manage the illness or injury in our absence; counselors assisting the patient and family in coping with emotional stress. We have an obligation to preserve and perpetuate these roles for the continued well-being of our profession and our clients.

The outcome audit focuses on the care that patients receive and has the potential for making an important impact if utilized properly. The onus of responsibility is on the professionals in home health care agencies to develop systematic means for exploiting this potential fully. The goal of such a review is not accumulation of impressive documents, but rather education and reeducation of the staff so that discrepancies are corrected and the quality of care is upgraded

PROCESS OF PATIENT CARE

Without an accurate understanding of the process of patient care, the outcome criteria would be almost impossible to achieve. A successful application of this process will almost always yield the accomplishment or achievement of the desired outcome.

The process of patient care is an orderly, systematic manner of determining the patient's problems, making plans to solve them, initiating the plan or assigning others to implement it, and evaluating the extent to which the plan was effective in resolving the problems identified.

1. *In-depth assessment with diagnoses*—identifies patient's health problems, the patient's capabilities to learn and to whom and at what level education must be directed.

2. *Goal planning with patient/family*—must involve patient/family to make them aware of care needed and understand that patient/family participation is expected.

   Long-term goals indicate knowledge, skills, and support necessary to assist patient to achieve personalized level of functioning.

   Short-term goals are written in order of priority for patient to accomplish by predetermined date.

3. *Implementation*—action taken on an individual level. Allows feedback for patient/family to digest newly acquired knowledge and skills.

4. *Evaluation*—documentation of action reflects the progress of care effectiveness and conclusions of intervention.

As a health care professional, documentation is one of the most important tasks performed. It is a method to demonstrate professional accountability and responsibility. Maintaining the clinical records play a key role in attesting to quality service:

A. Written evidence of all care given.

B. Means of communication to physician and to other disciplines.

C. Source of statistical data.

D. Compliance with state and federal guidelines.

E. Supports reimbursement.

Care plans are a vital part of a patient's record. They are a systematic, well-communicated, individual approach to patient care. The writing of a care plan entails an aggressive approach, placing the responsibility on the professional for initiating actions both for the writer and for others. The outcome criteria must be incorporated into the patient care plan to assure compliance with the established standards.

RECOMMENDED FORMS

1. Terms (see Fig. 2)

2. Outcome Criteria (see Fig. 3)

3. Data Summary (see Fig. 4)

4. Worksheet (Data Retrieval) (see Fig. 5)—Tool used for actual retrieval of criteria compliance. Compares actual performance to established criteria.

5. Audit Sumary and Evaluation (see Fig. 6)—Analyze variations to identify justifiable variations and true deficiencies and identify probable reasons for deficiencies.

Appropriate corrective action is described: how, by whom, by predetermined time. Such action is non-punitive, such as counseling, inservice education, patient education, staffing, policies, and procedures.

The Audit Summary and Evaluation is to be signed by the agency administrative officers to acknowledge accountability.

FIGURE 2
Terms

Target Population	Pertains to those patients who have a specific disease or condition for whom the criteria is developed.
Variables	Defined selected characteristics used to describe target population.
Criteria Subset	Organizational framework.
Outcome Criteria	Measurable standards of care to define patient's status at time of discharge.
Standards	Absolute goal. Each criterion should be achieved 100% of the time.
Exceptions	Element of criteria may be an unrealistic expectation, i.e., pre-existing condition.
	Straight line bracket means "such as." At least one of the elements should be found in the documentation.

FIGURE 3
Example of Outcome Criteria Form

OUTCOME CRITERIA

TARGET POPULATION _____   VARIABLES: A. _____
                  _____   B. _____
SERVICE: _____   C. _____

CRITERIA SUBSET	OUTCOME CRITERIA	STANDARDS	EXCEPTIONS

FIGURE 4
Example of Data Summary Form

DATA SUMMARY

AGENCY:_____ DATE:_____

NUMBER OF PATIENTS:_____ FROM:_____TO:_____

DIAGNOSIS:_____

EMPLOYEE NUMBER	PATIENT RECORD NUMBER *	1	2	3	4	5	6	7	8	9	10

*   EXPLANATION:

1. Number of total visits
2. Patient hospitalized immediately prior to admission to services (within 14 days)
3. Medical supervision (Private and Clinic)
4. Referred by (hospital, physician, nursing home, family, clinic)
5. Discharged to care of (family and self, significant other, hospital, nursing home, died)
6. All documentation-signed and dated
7. Nursing care plan recorded, revised, signed, and dated
8. Admission nursing assessment (physical and emotional)
9. Discharge nursing assessment (physical and emotional) or re-hospitalized
10. Sex, age

CODE SYMBOLS

✓ - Yes   Phy - Physician
X - No   SNF - Skilled Nursing Facility
P - Private   N/A - Non-Applicable
C - Clinic   S/C - Self-Care
H - Hospital S/O - Significant Other
F - Family   Fe - Female
D - Died   M   - Male

FIGURE 5
Example of Worksheet

WORKSHEET

SUMMARY OF CHART REVIEW   DATE:_____

TARGET POPULATION:_____

VARIABLES: a._____

             b._____

             c._____

OUTCOME CRITERIA

CHART ##	1	2	3	4	5	6	7	8	9	10	11	12	13	14	15	16	17	18	19	20
1.																				
2.																				
3.																				
4.																				
5.																				
6.																				
7.																				
8.																				
9.																				
10.																				
11.																				
12.																				
13.																				
14.																				
15.																				
16.																				
17.																				
18.																				
19.																				
20.																				
TOTALS																				
√																				
X																				
EX																				
ACTUAL PERFOR- MANCE %																				

FORMULA =   CODE SYMBOLS

√+ EX ÷ Total Number of Charts Reviewed X 100 =   √-CLEARLY MET
                                                               X-NOT MET
Actual Performance Percentage.   EX-MET BY EXCEPTION

FIGURE 6
Example of Audit Summary and Evaluation Form

AUDIT SUMMARY & EVALUATION

AGENCY: _____   DATE: _____

TARGET POPULATION: _____   VARIABLES: A. _____

TOTAL PATIENTS: _____   B. _____

COMMITTEE CHAIRPERSON: _____   C. _____

EXECUTIVE OFFICER: _____

OUTCOME CRITERIA	STANDARDS %	ACTUAL PERFORMANCE %	EVALUATION AND RECOMMENDATIONS

FIGURE 7
Example of Skilled Nursing Outcome Criteria

OUTCOME CRITERIA

TARGET POPULATION OPEN WOUND

SERVICE: SKILLED NURSING

VARIABLES: A. _____
B. _____
C. _____

CRITERIA SUBSET	OUTCOME CRITERIA	STANDARDS	EXCEPTIONS
Physical	1) Temperature is within 96 to 99°.	100%	Physician aware
	2) Healed wound.	100%	
	3) Skin surrounding wound intact and free of excoriation.	100%	
	4) Absence of pain at wound site.	100%	
	5) Describes oral intake of 1500-2000cc/daily with urinary output of clear amber urine.	100%	
Safety	6) No evidence of hazards: Scatter rugs Obstacles in walking path Inadequate lighting Outdated drugs	100%	
	7) Evidence of safety measures: Emergency plan and contact number Functional placement of furniture Siderails, if bedridden Proper storage of drugs	100%	
	Patient and/or significant other:		
Psycho-Social	8) Demonstrates acceptance of condition by willingness to resume lifestyle within physical limitations and abilities; including sexual activity.	100%	Pt. unwilling to discuss sexual activity.

Copyright, 1980
Florida Assoc.

FIGURE 7 (continued)

OUTCOME CRITERIA

TARGET POPULATION: _____ OPEN WOUND

CRITERIA SUBSET	OUTCOME CRITERIA	STANDARDS	EXCEPTIONS
Education	9) Describes medications as ordered: time, dosage, mode desired effects side effects complications-action to take	100%	
	10) Verbalizes knowledge of diet as ordered and menu planning.	100%	
	11) States signs and symptoms which necessitate medical advice: Increased tenderness, pain, inflammation, blanching, edema in operative area, temperature elevation.	100%	
	12) States plan for medical follow-up.	100%	
	13) Verbalizes knowledge of available Community Resources.	100%	

Colorado Quality Assurance Audit Criteria

Colorado Association of Home Health Agencies

Excerpted here is a rationale and examples for implementation of out-come audit criteria published by the Colorado Association of Home Health Agencies in 1983. Recognizing that reimbursement for care could be tied to outcome criteria, the Colorado Association provided a tool for retrospective record review for specific medical diagnoses or patient problems. Utilizing a process approach, the tool provides outcome measurement criteria to determine whether a patient's status is within acceptable ranges. The tool establishes a mechanism for recommendations and comments by the reviewer evaluating an individual case to facilitate concurrent development of a plan of care.

WHY OUTCOME CRITERIA?

The Advisory Committee for the Quality Assurance Program, Community Nursing Section, Colorado Department of Health developed "Process and Outcome Criteria: Background and Development," March 1980. This material, as well as a paper presented by Fran Adkins at the Home Health Agency Personnel Meeting, September 1980, was the basis for the audit development.

The use of outcome criteria assumes that (1) care affects the outcome of the patient's illness and influences the patient's future health status; and (2) identifiable outcomes exist that are primarily attributable to the care received. Outcome is defined as the alteration in health status of a patient that is the end result of care; a consequence or result. The use of outcome criteria for audit not only provides for the retrospective evaluation of care but a mechanism for the concurrent development of a patient plan of care. The criteria may be used to assess the patient, establish goals, and to evaluate progress toward those goals. Outcome criteria are also helpful in establishing patient teaching plans that include realistic goals and priorities.

In addition, outcome criteria can assist health professionals in communicating with patients, the public, and other groups. They help define the difference made by the provision of care. It is the hope of the committee that Medicare regulations and other reimbursement systems will be adjusted to consider this kind of care criteria as a basis for continued reimbursement. Reimbursement for care could be tied to outcome criteria.

This tool is a beginning step in defining quality skilled care. These audits have been tested by several home health agencies throughout Colorado and have been revised as a result of this testing. Those using the tool may find additional areas in which revision is needed.

The committee has made every effort to ensure that the audits are in accord with current recommendations and clinical practice at this time. However, in view of ongoing research and changes in clinical practice the user of these tools is urged to validate criteria using other current sources related to clincial practice.

AUDIT SHEET:
DIRECTIONS FOR COMPLETION AND USE

The audit analyzes each diagnosis or problem using the process approach of a specific discipline. It should be noted that either term, "patient" or "client," could be interchanged depending on the frame of reference with which one is reviewing the individual.

Each audit assumes that the specified diagnosis or problem is the only condition present. Multiple conditions indicate multiple audits for that individual. For example, if a patient with cancer is receiving chemotherapy and the prognosis is terminal, then the general cancer audit, chemotherapy audit and terminal care audit is implemented.

Topic: Diagnosis or problem to be evaluated for this particular patient/client.

Special note: Clarifying comments regarding the topic.

Criteria to be met:	100 percent unless otherwise stated.
Goal:	The purpose of the discipline in intervening with patient/client with this specific diagnosis/problem.
Process parameters:	The series of activities directed toward measurable assurances of comprehensive quality of care. The processes are physiological assessment, psychosocial/environmental assessment, evaluation of patient compliance with education and treatment, and the prevention of complications.
Outcome/goal:	Expected result of the intervention of the health care providers activity. Ideally the goals of care will be the outcomes of care.
Assessment parameters:	Objective and subjective areas to be evaluated in order to determine outcome/goal achievement.
Outcome measurement Criteria:	Explanation of the acceptable ranges of the assessment parameters, as defined by professional consensus.
Criteria met:	*Yes* column checked indicates that the criterion measure has been met.

No column checked indicates that the criterion measure has *not* been met, although it was expected.

Note: If a *no* answer is given there should be evidence of continuing care or the abnormal outcome protocol implemented.

N/A column checked indicates the criterion measure either "does not apply" or is inappropriate to measure for a given individual.

Note: If N/A column checked, documentation must exist in last column to substantiate its usage/exception; e.g., high blood pressure exists and is normal for patient due to presence of another disease process or circumstance, e.g., physical or mental disability, end-stage disease.

Continuing care criteria: An asterisk in this column indicates an outcome measurement criterion that *must* be met before services can appropriately be discontinued.

Criteria met: *Yes* column checked indicates that the criterion has been met.

No column checked indicates that the criterion has *not* been met, although it was expected.

Note: If a *no* answer is given there should be evidence of continuing care or an exception noted in the last column.

Abnormal outcome protocol: The problem solving process that must be documented whenever an outcome measurement criteria is NOT MET.

Recommendations and comments: Recording space for auditor's recommendations and comments.

Documentation of N/A: Documentation of N/As to substantiate exceptions.

PATIENT CARE AUDITS
NURSING TOPICS

1. Chronic intractable pain
2. Terminal care
3. Cancer—general
4. Immunology
5. Radiation therapy
6. Chemotherapy
7. Diabetes mellitus
8. Hypertension
9. Parkinson's disease
10. Multiple sclerosis
11. Cataract removal
12. Wounds/surgical traumatic
13. Wounds/decubitus ulcers
14. Colostomy
15. Ileostomy
16. Urinary diversion
17. Urinary tract infection
18. Chronic obstructive pulmonary disease
19. Pneumonia—respiratory infections
20. Post-pulmonary embolism
21. Laryngectomy
22. Tracheostomy
23. Peripheral vascular disease
24. Congestive heart failure
25. Post-myocardial infarction
26. Cerebral vascular accident with hemiplegia
27. Thrombophlebitis
28. Pernicious anemia
29. Rheumatoid arthritis
30. Degenerative joint disease (osteoarthritis)
31. Spinal cord injury
32. Closed head injury
33. Schizophrenic disorders
34. Neurotic or reactive depression
35. Psychotic depression—major affective disorder
36. Substance, drugs, and alcohol abuse

FIGURE 1

Explanation of Quality Audit Form

COLORADO QUALITY AUDIT FOR INDIVIDUAL CASE RECORD

Topic:
Special Note:
% Criteria to be Met: 100% unless otherwise stated
Recommended Readings:

Goal:

Nursing Process Parameter	Outcome Goal	Assessment Parameters	Outcome Measurement Criteria	Criteria Met Yes No N/A	Continuing Care Criteria	Criteria Met Yes No	Abnormal Outcome Protocol	Recommendations & Comments Documentation of N/A
Process activities include physiological assessment, psychosocial/environmental assessment, evaluation of compliance with education and treatment, and the prevention of complications.	Desired results of intervention: for example, for a patient with COPD, one of the goals is to stabilize respiratory status.	Specific areas that must be assessed to determine achievement of the outcome/goal. For example, dyspnea, sputum, pluse, etc., must be assessed to determine if the respiratory status is stabilized.	Measurements decide if the patient's/client's status is within acceptable ranges. These ranges are listed in this column. For example, the acceptable range for sputum is colorless, white or clear.	**Yes:** When this column is checked, outcome criteria have been met. **No:** When this column is checked, care continues or the abnormal outcome protocol is implemented. **N/A:** When this column is checked, documentation appears in last column.	Indicates a criteria that must be met before patient/client services can be discontinued.	**Yes:** When this column is checked, consider discharge/level of care change. **No:** When this column is checked, care continues or exception appears in last column.	Process to occur when the patient/client does not meet the acceptable range/measurement criteria and the goal is not met.	Auditor's comments/recomendation and documentation of exceptions to the criteria.

FIGURE 2
Example of Completed Quality Audit Form

COLORADO QUALITY AUDIT FOR INDIVIDUAL CASE RECORD

Topic: Wounds/Decubitis
Special Note: #13
Recommended Readings: Broadwell, Debra C., and Bettie S. Jackson, *Principles of Ostomy Care*, The C. V. Mosby Company, St. Louis, 1982, pp. 687-710.
Lippincott Manual of Nursing Practice, 3rd Edition, J. B. Lippincott Co., Philadelphia, 1982, pp. 64-67.
% Criteria to be Met: 100% Unless otherwise stated
Goal: Curing of disease process.

Nursing Process Parameter	Outcome Goal	Assessment Parameters	Outcome Measurement Criteria	Criteria Met Yes	Criteria Met No	Criteria Met N/A	Continuing Care Criteria	Criteria Met Yes	Criteria Met No	Abnormal Outcome Protocol	Recommendations & Comments Documentation of N/A
Physiological assessment	Healed wounds	S: Pain/Discomfort	None							Document	
		O: BP	90-160/60-90							Report to physician and team	
		T	96.4°-99°F/35.8°-37.2°C orally				*				
		P	60-90 regular								
		R	16-20, at rest, unlabored								
		Ulcer site(s) appearance	Healed/Eschar may be present				*			Review treatment and compliance factor	
		Drainage	None				*				
		Swelling/induration	No undue swelling or induration				*			Develop and implement new care plan	
		Color	No undue color changes				*				
		Temperature	No undue changes in temperature at site				*				
Psychosocial environmental assessment	Acceptance of treatment program Family/significant others coping with patient illness	Coping ability	Verbalizes understanding of treatment course and complies with program. Effective communication with the health team.							Seek consultation	
		Involvement of others	Maintains caring, stable relationships Relies appropriately on care givers for assistance								

Nursing Process Parameter	Outcome Goal	Assessment Parameters	Outcome Measurement Criteria	Criteria Met Yes	No	N/A	Continuing Care Criteria	Criteria Met Yes	No	Abnormal Outcome Protocol	Recommendations & Comments Documentation of N/A
		Physical Environment	Is established to promote wound healing (devices to aid circulation; e.g., padding, appropriate bed or mattress, etc.)								
Evaluation of compliance with education and treatment	Medication compliance	Medication Intake/understanding	Teaching and verbalized understanding recorded							Same	
			Taking medication/achieving therapeutic effect								
			Verbalizes signs and symptoms and what to report/treat								
	Treatment compliance	Ulcer management	Measures taken to reduce pressure, improve circulation and prevent contamination								
			Maintained sterility and integrity of dressing (if present)								
			Verbalizes/demonstrates proper technique and S&S of complications								
	Nutritional compliance	Diet/hydration	Intake is high protein, high carbohydrate, high vitamin C diet and drinks 2+ liters of fluid/day (unless contraindicated)								

FIG. 2 (continued)

Nursing Process Parameter	Outcome Goal	Assessment Parameters	Outcome Measurement Criteria	Criteria Met Yes	No	N/A	Continuing Care Criteria	Continuing Criteria Met Yes	No	Abnormal Outcome Protocol	Recommendations & Comments Documentation of N/A
	Activity compliance	Activity	Activity promotes ulcer healing by increasing circulation Compliance with restrictions								
	Resource management	Medical appointment	Appointments kept								
		Community resources	Is aware of community resources (American Cancer Society, home health agencies, etc.) and how to get help and supplies as needed Uses appropriately								
Prevention of complications	Absence of complications	Chronic pain Infection (local or systemic) Failure to heal Amyloidosis Severe malnutrition and wasting	Asymptomatic Knows complications and preventive measures Knows where, when, and how to get help				*			When these occur, reassess in depth from the beginning of this audit	

Contributors: Denver Visiting Nurse Service and Northeast Colorado Visiting Nurse Service. Revised May 1983. © Colorado Home Health Care Standards Committee.

Part 5

Discipline-Specific Approaches

Outcome Criteria for Physical Therapy, Speech Pathology, and Occupational Therapy

Florida Association of Home Health Agencies

This excerpt and the one that follows from the Visiting Nurse Association of Dallas, give examples of outcome standards for allied health professions. The Florida outcome audit described in Part 4 is taken a step further in the examples given here by specifying outcome criteria for physical therapy (Fig. 1), speech pathology (Fig. 2), and occupational therapy (Fig. 3). The Visiting Nurse Association of Dallas provides social work standards and outcomes for clients.

Reprinted with permission from *The Florida Association of Home Health Agencies, Inc., Presents a Quality Assurance Program,* 2nd ed., copyright © 1980, and *Occupational Therapy Addendum,* copyright © 1983, Florida Association of Home Health Agencies, Inc., Tallahassee.

FIGURE 1
Example of Physical Therapy Outcome Criteria

OUTCOME CRITERIA

TARGET POPULATION   CVA   VARIABLES: A. _____

                                            B. _____

SERVICE: PHYSICAL THERAPY   C. _____

CRITERIA SUBSET	OUTCOME CRITERIA	STANDARDS	EXCEPTIONS
Physical	Patient shall have achieved:	100%	Pain not amenable to treatment.
	1. Reduction of pain to tolerable levels.		No pain
	2. Sufficient range in involved extremity to permit bathing and dressing.	100%	
	3. At least reflex function in involved extremity. (ability to stiffen LE for ambulation).	100%	Flexion withdrawal reflex. Flail U.E.
	4. Reduction of edema to minimum or zero.		
Functional	Patient demonstrates independently or with minimal assistance:		

	5. Bed mobility activities
	    rolling
	    scooting
	    sitting
		100%	

	6. Transfer activities
	    Bed to chair
	    Chair to commode
	    Chair to car
		100%	Lacks potential

	7. Personal hygiene activities
	    Bathing
	    Dressing
	    Feeding
		100%	Lacks potential

	8. Ambulation indoors and out with or without assistive device:	100%	Lacks potential

FIG. 1 (continued)

OUTCOME CRITERIA

TARGET POPULATION: _____ CVA

CRITERIA SUBSET	OUTCOME CRITERIA	STANDARDS	EXCEPTIONS

	9. Ascending and descending, with or without assistive device.
	   stairs
	   steps
	   curb
		100%	Lacks potential

Safety	Patient and/or significant other demonstrates:
	
	10. Evidence of safety measures:
	   Grab bars
	   Adaptive equipment
	   Non-slip surfaces in
	    bathroom
	    tub
	   Adequate lighting
	   Functional placement of furniture
	   Handrails
	   No scatter rugs
	   No polished floors
	   No obstacles in pathway
		100%	

	11. Awareness of sensory deficits:
	   routine skin inspection
	   protection of affected extremity
	   avoidance of extreme temperatures on involved
	   extremity.
		100%	

Education	12. Knowledge of use and care of all equipment- where to call for repairs and maintenance.	100%	
	13. Plan for medical follow-up.	100%	
	14. Knowledge of community resources.	100%	
	15. Home exercise program.	100%	

FIGURE 2
Example of Speech Pathology Outcome Criteria

OUTCOME CRITERIA

TARGET POPULATION PARKINSON'S DISEASE   VARIABLES: A. _____

                                                                B. _____

SERVICE: _SPEECH PATHOLOGY_   C. _____

CRITERIA SUBSET	OUTCOME CRITERIA	STANDARDS	EXCEPTIONS
I. IMPAIRMENT			I. IMPAIRMENT
A. Motor Speech	1. Pt. demonstrates ability to produce intelligible speech.	100%	Presence of co-existing sensory, medical, or coping deficits. Illiteracy
1. Respiration	2. Pt. demonstrates breathing pattern for speech.	100%	
2. Phonation	3. Pt. demonstrates voluntary control over phonation.	100%	
	4. Pt. demonstrates voluntary control of voice intensity level.	100%	
3. Articulation	5. Pt. demonstrates coordination and precision of lips, tongue, and jaw movement.	100%	
	6. Pt. demonstrates ability to articulate isolated consonants and vowels.	100%	
	7. Pt. demonstrates balanced nasality.	100%	
B. Graphic	8. Pt. demonstrates ability to communicate through writing.	100%	

FIG. 2 (continued)

OUTCOME CRITERIA

TARGET POPULATION: PARKINSON'S DISEASE

CRITERIA SUBSET	OUTCOME CRITERIA	STANDARDS	EXCEPTIONS
I. SAFETY	9. Pt. and/or significant other indicates awareness of an emergency plan.	100%	
I. PSYCHO-SOCIAL	10. Pt. demonstrates intention to maintain present lifestyle.	100%	
V. EDUCATION	11. Pt. and/or significant other verbalizes knowledge of how disease process affects speech.	100%	
	12. Pt. and/or significant other verbalizes intention to comply with home program.		

FIGURE 3
Example of Occupational Therapy Outcome Criteria

OUTCOME CRITERIA

TARGET POPULATION: CARDIAC (MYOCARDIAL INFARCTION)   PAGE ___1___

CRITERIA SUBSET	OUTCOME CRITERIA	STANDARDS	EXCEPTIONS

PHYSICAL	1. Patient will demonstrate ability to resume ADL's without shortness of breath or angina pain:
	  feeding
	  dressing
	  bathing
	  grooming
	  light housekeeping
		100%	Medical instability

FUNCTIONAL	Patient demonstrates: 2. Proper body mechanics 3. Work simplification techniques 4. Energy conservation techniques	100% 100% 100%	

SAFETY	Patient and/or significant other shall demonstrate:
	5. Evidence of safety measures
	  emergency plan
	  smoke detector
	  no scatter rugs or slippery floors
	  non-obstructive furniture placement
	  adequate lighting and ventilation
	  grab bars
	  shower chair
	  rubber bath mats and/or non-slip strips
		100%	

FIG. 3 (continued)

OUTCOME CRITERIA

TARGET POPULATION: CARDIAC (MYOCARDIAL INFARCTION)

CRITERIA SUBSET	OUTCOME CRITERIA	STANDARDS	EXCEPTIONS

PSYCHOSOCIAL	6. Patient verbalizes that he has successfully planned and executed activities within scope of tolerance
	    ADL
	    leisure time
	    sexual activity
		100%	

EDUCATION	Patient and/or significant other shall demonstrate: 7. Knowledge and understanding of cardiac condition and precautions 8. Ability to monitor pulse rate in relation to activity 9. Knowledge of relaxation techniques 10. Home program 11. Plan for medical follow-up 12. Knowledge of community resources	100% 100% 100% 100% 100% 100%	

MSW Standards and Outcomes for Clients

Visiting Nurse Association of Texas

MSW PROTOCOL

The standards and norms created by the Visiting Nurse Association consist of problems that were felt to be commonly encountered by the group as a whole and problems specific to the homebound disabled and aged who comprise the target population. Because of the clients' decreased independence, family members and significant others must become operative in problem solution, thus necessitating the family-centered approach. Because of the latter, it is emphasized that oftentimes the MSW, although receiving a referral on a specific client, must and does deal with any additional psychosocial problems occurring within the family as a whole in as much as those problems impinge upon the client's health. As such, it was an extremely difficult task to pinpoint the modal time frame of MSW service, on even the simplest problem developed, and thus the ranges indicated in the projected units of service were purposely selected to accommodate the individual variations attributable to initial levels of functioning, discrepancies in problem perception, adequacy of support systems, and temporal intervening variables.

Reprinted with permission of the Visiting Nurse Association of Texas, Dallas, Texas, 1980.

Lastly, a number of problems defined by the MSWs have also been defined by nursing and are dealt with by both professions with the same goals in mind. However, these goals may or may not be reached through different types of interactions.

A partial listing of diagnoses follows.

Health Problem Diagnosis	Projected Client Outcomes	Acceptable Client Outcomes
1. Coping abilities, impairment of		
a. Inability to identify stress factors.	1. Client/family verbally acknowledge state when in stress.	1. 85%
	2. Client/family able to state cause of stress.	2. 50%
	3. Client/family identify times of low stress.	3. 85%
b. Inability to identify options for relief of stress situation.	1. Client/family behaviorally acknowledge the existing stress situation.	1. 85%
	2. Client/family verbally acknowledge the stress situation.	2. 70%
	3. Client/family verbally acknowledge the need for relief.	3. 70%
	4. Client/family utilize own resources for the alleviation of stress.	4. 40%
	5. Client/family explore and initiate multiple extrafamilial alternatives.	5. 60%
2. Depression (typified by a negative world view, past, present, and/or future; disturbances in eating and/or sleeping; withdrawal; frequent crying; agitation; low energy level; feelings of hopelessness; numerous somatic complaints)	1. Client/family acknowledge depressive behaviors.	1. 95%
	2. Client/family acknowledge that the behaviors are symptomatic of depression.	2. 70%
	3. Client/family attribute depression to trauma or loss.	3. 60%
	4. Client/family express feelings associated with depression.	4. 70%
	5. Client/family acknowledge resolution is possible.	5. 60%
	6. Client/family identify strengths, remaining coping skills, and resources.	6. 75%
	7. Client/family identify alternatives for problem resolution.	7. 60%
3. Inability to utilize community resources.	1. Client/family acknowledge existence of problem that could be ameliorated with aid from community resource.	1. 100%
	2. Client/family acknowledge inability to utilize resources.	2. 80%
	3. Client/family explore availability of appropriate community resources.	3. a. With assistance, 75% b. Without assistance, 60%
	4. Client/family initiate contact with appropriate resources.	4. a. With assistance, 60% b. Without assistance, 40%
	5. Client/family follow through with utilizing resources.	5. a. With assistance, 40% b. Without assistance, 30%
	6. Client/family continue to utilize community resources when similar situations arise.	6. a. With assistance, 50% b. Without assistance, 25%

Quality Assurance
in Public Health

Margaret McWilliams Kline, Mary Lee Tracy
and Sharon Davis Howell

Recognizing that programs based entirely on federal and state guidelines were inadequate to demonstrate the outcomes of patient care at the local level, the Office of Nursing in Georgia's Department of Human Resources applied the concepts of the American Nurses' Association Quality Assurance Model to community health nursing. The marked improvement in documentation that resulted from the peer review audit demonstrates the advantages of utilizing the existing expertise of public health nurses in practice settings.

Georgia's Department of Human Resources (DHR) has the awesome task of planning and providing quality community health services to 4.5 million people in 159 counties. These counties are organized into ten health districts with nine additional sub-units each using individual approaches to solving their unique health problem. In addition, each county has its own health department, many of these with satellite centers. There is great diversity in size, population, and resources among the counties: some large metropolitan

Reprinted from *Nursing & Health Care,* 4 (November 1980), copyright © 1980, National League for Nursing, pp. 192–196, 207.
Public health and community health are used synonymously in this paper.

counties have over a million people, rapid transit, and complex medical centers; by contrast, an adjacent county of 2,000 population may have no public transportation and only the services of one community health nurse.

PROBLEM-ORIENTED RECORD CHOSEN

Georgia began applying the American Nurses' Association Quality Assurance concepts to community health nursing when a group of nurses recognized that quality assurance could make an important contribution to successful health programs.[1] The initial application of these concepts came in the development and implementation of a problem-oriented record (POR) system. The nurses realized that a POR system would provide a framework for specificity and clarity previously unknown in recording the interaction of the health services and the communities they serve.

A statewide committee was organized with 12 representatives from the various levels of community health nursing. This committee endorsed a system very much in line with that recommended by Dr. Lawrence Weed.[2] After trial uses and subsequent revisions, DHR Health District 8, Unit 1, the Valdosta District, volunteered to serve as a test area for the newly developed system. The step by step implementation of POR will be described later in this article.

With the reorganization of the record-keeping activity came the need for nurses to conduct their recording in a more organized manner. This led to questioning what exactly was being done for clients entering one or more of the eleven health programs. A State Standards of Care Steering Committee, which was composed of nurses and nutritionists, was the natural consequence. This committee selected five main program areas for which standards of care would be written. To a large extent, the material was already available in program manuals, so the subcommittee, activity centered on applying the ANA concepts of standards of care to this content.

Two years later, the Georgia State Standards of Care for Public Health Nursing were printed and distributed to the 159 counties and district offices.[3] Currently, the state is in the process of implementing these 68 standards.

MODEL FOR QUALITY ASSURANCE

The ANA Quality Assurance Model (Table 1) involves seven steps. The first two were implemented by the activities described above.

Measurement was the third step. Several of the program units already had definitive audit activity and a few districts had conducted record audits and peer reviews. The State Office of Nursing has as its next goal the development of a common audit tool coordinated with the standards of care and the existing program audit tool.

TABLE 1
Model for Quality Assurance: Implementation of Standards

1. Identify values.

2. Identify structure, process and outcome standards and criteria.

3. Measurements needed to determine degree of attainment of criteria and standards.

4. Make interpretations about strengths and weaknesses based upon measurements.

5. Identify possible courses of action.

6. Choose course of action.

7. Take action.

Reprinted with permission from *Guidelines for Review of Nursing Care at the Local Level* (Kansas City, MO: American Nurses' Association, 1976), p. 11.

Step four in the ANA model had been partially addressed from the beginning of this process and, as anticipated, obvious weaknesses were identified. Interpretation of the weaknesses led to the diagnosis that the role of our 750 generalized public health nurses was expanded before they were optimally prepared.

ROLE EXPANSION

In 1975, we began developing, with the cooperation of seven baccalaureate schools of nursing, a continuing education workshop titled Basic Skills in Health Appraisal. This workshop prepares our nurses to do the early and periodic screening, diagnosis, and treatment (EPSDT) assessments. Preparation takes place in two phases: (1) a 14-day didactic/laboratory practice session; (2) a three-month preceptorship, during which six complete assessments are recorded, using POR, and submitted to the nursing faculty for critique. A Women's Health Workshop and an Adult Health Workshop are also being offered to the generalized public health nurse to assist her into the expanded role.

The workshops are illustrations of how we have implemented the ANA Model for Quality Assurance Steps 4, 5, 6, and 7 in this one area, i.e., meeting educational needs. The general audit tool when implemented will, of course, identify many other needs for improvement.

Development of the quality assurance system thus far clearly indicates the degree of dedication of our Georgia public health nurses to the concepts of quality assurance which we are confident will provide our citizens with better quality health care at the local level.

IMPLEMENTING ONE COMPONENT

The process of implementing quality assurance components at the local level is illustrated by describing activities of the nursing staff in the Valdosta District. This district of ten counties began by providing the test site for full scale POR implementation (see Figs. 1-5 for basic forms and instructions used in teaching the POR method). Changing from a source-oriented record to a highly structured problem-oriented record is a traumatic experience when superimposed upon an active health department.

Initially, the new system of record keeping was viewed with real anxiety. Inservice education was provided by a district coordinator of nursing service on an individual and group basis, in an atmosphere in which questions and concerns were encouraged until the staff was able to use procedures and terminology with greater ease. In addition, a state-wide convention was held to gather nurses from all service units together for training.

Literature explaining the rationale and methodology for problem-oriented recording was available, and staff members were provided with an adjustment period which lasted approximately two years. The inevitable mistakes were made without fear of embarassment or reprimands, and in time the staff members became skillful in the use of problem-oriented recording and developed a positive attitude about its benefit.

It soon became apparent that the entire record management system needed an overhaul. A new policy was developed and implemented with all client records centralized in a single record room. A clerk was selected from the department, was oriented and, was placed in charge, monitoring distribution, temporary location of, and return of each family record. Record conversion was accomplished by nurses as clients were scheduled for service.

Inservice education programs continued to deal with the whole spectrum of quality assurance. From this broad approach, the staff was guided to focus first on the family planning program. Discussions included changes in scientific technology and its impact on nursing care, values placed on family planning services by clients, client acceptance of services provided by family planning nursing specialists, development and use of protocols, and standards of nursing practice governing provision of services. In addition, content teaching about the federal and state guidelines governing provision of family planning services took place. Elements of care mandated by these regulations were recognized as constituting a base on which a more comprehensive program for quality assurance could be constructed. The nursing staff recognized that a program based entirely on federal and state guidelines was inadequate and considered these guidelines only as an expedient nucleus around which a comprehensive program could be later developed.

WRITING STANDARDS

The Standard of Care format as developed by Wilfong et al.,[4] was adapted by the Georgia State Quality Assurance Steering Committee as the pattern for constructing standards of care. The Valdosta District used this same format to write their Family Planning Standards of Care for nine categories identifying outcome, process, and screening criteria; critical time, standard, exceptions, resources, and best location for the information in the problem-oriented record (see Fig. 6).

Of these categories, the generation of process and outcome criteria was described by the staff as difficult, tedious, and time consuming. Meticulous attention was required to ferret out appropriate material for outcome, process, and screening criteria. Critical time was determined using professional judgment, federal and state regulations. Consistent with the ANA Guidelines, the critical time was set at 100 percent so that all cases not meeting this standard would be examined.

MEASURING SUCCESS

The next step was to determine the degree of attainment of the standard. The district audit committee met on a quarterly basis to review the county record audits using a tool developed by the district with audits forwarded to the district chief of nursing and her assistant.

Staff members reported initial feelings of anxiety about being audited by peers, but simultaneously reported a marked improvement in the quality of documentation of services provided to patients. It took six months for the majority of staff to report that they were comfortable with the audit procedures and considered the process beneficial to the improvement of practice. As an example of the process involved at this level, the assistant director of nursing reported that a recent audit pinpointed a lack of documentation of the history of patient's problems with contraception. The ANA advised that, when strengths and weaknesses of the nursing practice have been identified, action can be taken to reinforce strengths and to reduce weaknesses. Consequently, special inservice education was scheduled to improve the documentation of patient histories. ANA stresses that each time actions are taken, the progress of nursing practice needs to be reassessed and remeasured.

FIGURE 1
Individual History Data Base

Georgia Department of Human Resources·

⁴² INDIVIDUAL HISTORY DATA BASE

Target Population: Female Patients in Family Planning Clinics

43-Name	44-Date	45-Address	46-Phone

47-Reason For Visit

Pregnancy Prevention

48-Past History: Illnesses, Hospitalization, Trauma, Allergies, Habits

In addition to general history:

Obstetrical History should include number of full-term children, pre-
mature births, abortions, and living children as well as any complications of pregnancy, labor, delivery and post-partum period. The date
of menarche; frequency, regularity, length of menses, and date of last
menstrual period should be obtained.
Sexual History should include frequency of intercourse, number of
partners, and problems.
Habits should include use of alcohol, drugs, tobacco.

49-Family History: Heart Disease, Cancer, Stroke, Diabetes, Allergies, Tuberculosis, Mental Illness, Rheumatic Fever, Kidney Disease, Hypertension

In addition to general history:

Family History should include any signficant illnesses, diseases,
or congenital abnormalities.

50-Dietary History: Food Habits, Therapeutic Diets, 24 hour recall, Food Resources

24-hour recall should be done on all patients on admission visit.

Food Resources should include Food Stamps, WIC.

51-Current Medications: Over the Counter and Prescription

Should be completed on all patients on admission visit and updated
on each follow-up visit.

If on no medications, state - None.

52-Sources of Health Care and Phone	53-Pharmacy Name and Phone
Primary physician	

54-Examiner's Name

·Use Back of Form For Additional Information Using Identifying Number.

Form 3048 (Rev. 1-77)

FIGURE 2
Problem List

Georgia Department of Human Resources

Target Population: ⁷³ PROBLEM LIST

Target Population: Female Patients in Family Planning Clinics

FAMILY NAME:					
75 DATE	76 NAME	77 PROBLEM NUMBER	78	PROBLEM	79 DATE OF Resolution
		1	Pregnancy prevention		
			(preventive health area of concern)		
			Other areas of concern or problems		
			identified should be added to the problem		
			list as they are identified.		
			Plans or referrals to agency programs		
			or community resources should be written		
			in progress notes rather than on problem		
			list.		

Form 3051 (Rev. 1-77)   (Over)

FIGURE 3
Individual Physical Data Base

GEORGIA DEPARTMENT OF HUMAN RESOURCES

55 **INDIVIDUAL PHYSICAL DATA BASE**

Target Population: Fema
Patients in Family
Planning Clinics.

56 Name			57 Date	58 Address		59 Phone
60 Birthdate	61 Height	62 Weight	63 Temperature	64 Pulse	65 Resp.	66 Blood Pressure - Sitting
			NE	NE	NE	Systolic Diastolic

67 Normal = ✓ Abnormal = x Not Evaluated = N.E.	68 Briefly Describe Significant Findings

69   SKIN ☐
— Color   — Nails
— Moisture   — Hair
— Texture   — Other
Pigment

HEAD – EYES ☐
— Acuity   — Pupils
— Conjunctiva — Red reflex
— Fontanelle   — Sclera
— Fundi   — Size
— Lids   — Tension
— Movement   — Other

EARS ☐
— Drums   — Mastoid
— Hearing   — Other _____

NOSE ☐
— Airways   — Transillumination
— Mucosa   — Other
— Septum

MOUTH ☐
— Breath   — Tongue
— Lips   — Salivary Ducts
— Teeth   — Speech
— Gums   — Other

THROAT ☐
— Tonsils   — Other
— Pharynx

NECK ☐
— Carotids   — Trachea
— Thyroid   — Other
— Neck veins

LYMPH NODES ☐
— Cervical   — Inguinal
— Occipital   — Epitrochlear
— Supraclavicular — Other
— Axillary

CHEST ☐
— Shape   — Respirations
— Symmetry   — Other

BREAST ☐
— Symmetry   — Other
— Nipples

HEART ☐
— Apical Impulse — Sounds S_1
— Rate S_2
— Rhythm   — Other

LUNGS ☐
— Fremitus   — Spoken voice
— Percussion   — Whispered voice
— Breath sounds — Other _____

BLOOD VESSELS' ☐
— Pulses   — Other

All systems are to be evaluated. Any
abnormal or unusual findings should be
described in the space provided.

If a system or parameter in a system is
not evaluated, this should be noted.

Form 3044   (Rev. 11-78)   (Over)

FIG. 3 (continued)

55   **INDIVIDUAL PHYSICAL DATA BASE**

67 Normal = ✓ Not Evaluated = N.E. Abnormal = x	68 Briefly Describe Significant Findings

69   **ABDOMEN**   ☐
 ___ Contour   ___ Liver
 ___ Peristalsis   ___ Kidneys
 ___ Spleen   ___ Other _____
     GENITALIA – MALE   ☐
 ___ Penis   ___ Testes
 ___ Scrotum   ___ Other _____
     GENITALIA – FEMALE   ☐
 ___ External   ___ Uterus
 ___ Vagina   ___ Adnexa
 ___ Cervix   ___ Other _____
     RECTAL   ☐
 ___ Sphincter   ___ Feces
 ___ Masses   ___ Other _____
 ___ Prostate
 BONES – JOINTS – MUSCLES   ☐
 ___ Muscle Strength   ___ Other _____
 ___ Range of motion
     EXTREMITIES   ☐
 ___ Color   ___ Other _____
     NEUROLOGICAL   ☐
 ___ Motor   ___ Sensory
 ___ Coordination .   ___ Gait
 ___ Reflexes   ___ Other _____
	It is recommended that a brief description of the uterus be written so that a comparison can be made with future exams.

70 Laboratory: Hematocrit, Urinalysis, Special Studies

    Hematocrit
    Urinalysis
    VDRL
    GC Culture
    Pap Smear

71 Treatment Plan

    See initial progress notes.

72 Examiner's Name:

Form 3044 (Rev. 11-78)   (Reverse Side)

FIGURE 4
Family Planning Flow Sheet

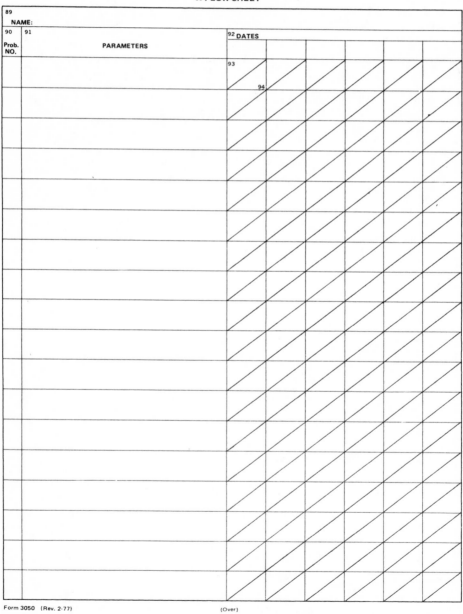

Georgia Department of Human Resources
88 **FLOW SHEET**

Form 3050 (Rev. 2-77)   (Over)

FIGURE 5
Progress Notes

Georgia Department of Human Resources

80PROGRESS NOTES

81 Page No. _____

Target Population: Female Patients in Family Planning Clinics

82 FAMILY NAME:				
83 DATE	84 NAME	85 Prob. NO.	86 SOAP	87 NOTES
				Initial progress notes should include:
				S - (1) brief social history; demographic data, such as directions to home (if needed), home phone number or phone number of a relative or neighbor.
				(2) Other pertinent information related by patient or family member.
				O - See Flow Sheet, History and Physical Data Base (it is not necessary to repeat in this section information that is recorded on these forms.)
				A - Interpretation of subjective and objective findings (should document that individual is a normal female requesting family planning services; a high-risk patient requiring special follow-up; or is a poor candidate for a specific contraceptive method.)
				P - Diagnostic Tests other than laboratory (ex. PPD)
				Therapeutic 1. SBE Taught 2. Contraceptive method initiated 3. Routine family planning care plans 4. Follow-up clinic appointment
				Educational 1. Informed consent obtained. 2. Health care instructions/counselling appropriate for this individual.
				Follow-up progress notes should indicate progress made toward achieving initial plans; revision of plans, identification of other problems and plans for these identified problems; discharge information, etc.

Form 3046 (Rev. 2-77)   (Over)

FIGURE 6
Family Planning Standards of Care

COMPONENT: FAMILY PLANNING		Office of Nursing
VARIABLES: 1. Initial visit		Department of Human Resources
2. Annual visit		—Physical Health
3. Change of method		Atlanta, Georgia

TARGET POPULATION:
Women Age 10 - 44

Outcomes	Process	Screening Criteria	Critical Time	Standard	Exception	Resource	Record
Optimum total health and awareness of risks and benefits related to contraceptive use.	1. Relevant history (patient & family) identified and recorded, including: 1.1 Previous method (include type)/duration of use 1.2 Last menstrual period 1.3 Age at which periods began 1.4 Irregular periods or amenorrhea 1.5 Pelvic pain/painful periods/abdominal pain 1.6 Unexplained or excessive vaginal bleeding 1.7 Past problems with contraceptives 1.8 Symptoms of pregnancy 1.9 Vaginal discharge or pelvic infection 1.10 Chest pain 1.11 Blurring or fading of vision 1.12 Severe headaches 1.13 Depression or irritability 1.14 Thromboembolic disease 1.15 Phlebitis/varicose veins/leg pains 1.16 Breast mass/breast discharge/breast surgery 1.17 Asthma or drug allergy 1.18 Full term/prem./abortion/live now 1.19 Complications of pregnancy or delivery 1.20 Significant illnesses, hospitalizations, or	1. Patient requests Family Planning services	1. First visit, annual visit, and as otherwise indicated.	1. 100%	1. None	1. 6, 8, 9, 11, 12	Data Base I Problem List FP Flow Sheet FP Visit Form Progress Notes

FIG. 6 (continued)

Outcomes	Process	Screening Criteria	Critical Time	Standard	Exception	Resource	Record
	responses listed to in-dicated systems review)						
	1.21 Heart, liver (jaundice), or kidney disease.						
	1.22 Diabetes (or abnormal blood or urine sugar)						
	1.23 High blood pressure or stroke						
	1.24 Pelvic tumor (fibroids or cancer, etc.)						
	1.25 Anemia, clotting or bruising problems						
	1.26 Significant diseases in family						
	1.27 VD history						
	1.28 Fever						
	2. Counseling and education on all methods (group and/or individual) including "B.R.A.I.D.E.D."	2. Patient makes decision regarding choice of method with knowledge of potential risk factors	2. First visit or if change of method	2. 100%	2. None	2. Same as above	
	3. Collection and recording of relevant physical findings	3. Clinical findings are within normal limits	3. First visit and annual visit	3. 100%	3. None	3. Same as above	
	3.1 Laboratory						
	3.11 Weight/height						
	3.12 Blood pressure						
	3.13 Hematocrit/Pap smear						
	3.14 Pregnancy test/gonorrhea culture/VDRL (if indicated)					DHEW Stan-dard	
	3.15 Urinalysis						
	3.2 Physical						
	3.21 Thyroid						
	3.22 Breast and axilla						
	3.23 Heart/lungs (if respiratory symptoms present)						
	3.24 Skin/hair/complexion						
	3.25 Abdomen						
	3.26 Pelvic						
	3.27 Rectal/vaginal						
	3.28 Extremities						

FIG. 6 (continued)

Outcomes	Process	Screening Criteria	Critical Time	Standard	Exception	Resource	Record
	3.29 IUD strings visible 3.30 Breast self-exam taught 4. Post-interview and teaching regarding selected method	4. Patient demonstrates understanding by: 4.1 Keeping follow-up appointments 4.2 Using clinic regimen 4.3 Desribing use effectiveness of method chosen 4.4 Listing danger signs and possible complications 4.5 Enumerating side effects 4.6 Where applicable, describing care of method	4. First visit and as indicated	4. 100%	4. Inadequate	4. Same as above	Informed consent form
	Refills						
	5. Patient/family history updated and recorded 5.1 Oral contraceptives his torical 1.1, 1.2, 1.4-1.17, 1.20-1.27 5.2 IUD historical components listed from above 1.1 - 1.6, 1.8, 1.9, 1.20, 1.27, 1.28 5.3 Diaphragm historical components listed from above 1.1, 1.2, 1.4 - 1.6, 1.8, 1.9	5. Patient desires to continue method	5. As indicated 5.1 Initial visit at 3 months then every 3-6 months 5.2 Initial, at 1 month, to 3 months, then annual 5.3 1 week, to 3 months, then annual	5. 100%	5. None	5. Same as above	

The district audit committee continually reevaluates policies and procedures while simultaneously reviewing the documentation process and the individual nurse's performance pattern to ascertain problems with the system or staff. The findings are discussed by the committee and then corrective measures prescribed.

SUMMARY

The implementation of the quality assurance program is spreading across the state. The process is slow, but state and district nursing leaders are confident that steady progress is being made in providing Georgia's community health nurses with the tools they need for quality care in their expanded role.

ABOUT THE AUTHORS

Margaret M. Kline, MN, RN, is Nursing Program Specialist, Office of Nursing, Division of Public Health, Georgia Department of Human Resources, Atlanta. Mary Lee Tracy, MN, RN, was a degree candidate in the masters program at Emory University, Atlanta, Georgia, when this work took place. Sharon Davis Howell, MPH, RN, is District Clinical Coordinator, Clayton County Health Department, Georgia.

REFERENCES

1. *Guidelines for Review of Nursing Care at the Local Level* (Kansas City, MO: American Nurses' Association, 1976).

2. Lawrence L. Weed, *Medical Records, Medical Education and Patient Care.* (Cleveland, OH: Case Western Reserve University Press, 1969).

3. *State Standards of Care for Public Health Nursing* (Atlanta: Georgia Department of Human Resources, Division of Physical Health, Office of Nursing, 1979).

4. Marilyn Wilfong, et al., "Starting a System for Evaluating Quality of Care: Process and Product," *American Journal of Maternal Child Nursing* (May/June, 1976).

A Client Classification System Adaptable for Computerization

Karen Martin

This article provides a description of the patient classification system developed by the Visiting Nurses Association of Omaha, which addressed patient problems encountered by nurses in the community health setting. Specifying four categories in which nursing interventions occur, the Omaha VNA developed expected outcome and criteria schemes based on identified nursing problems and clusters of descriptions. Utilizing a family-centered approach, the classification scheme provides nurses and community health agencies with a tool to improve delivery, documentation, and description of patient care.

Providing, documenting, and describing client care are never simple tasks. The 1960s and 70s were a period of extraordinary growth for the Visiting Nurses Association of Omaha (VNA) in Nebraska. Both the increasing size and the complexity of the VNA necessitated changes in the method of documentation in order to overcome staff frustration.

Reprinted with permission from *Nursing Outlook*, 30 (November-December 1982), copyright
© 1982, American Journal of Nursing Company, pp. 515-517.
The project was supported by contracts (No. 231-75-0818 and 231-77-0068) with the Division
of Nursing, U.S. Department of Health and Human Services.

The VNA's 150 employees serve individuals, families, and groups of all ages in the urban areas of Omaha and also the rural areas of Douglas and Sarpy counties. Programs available to the 500,000 population include home care of the sick, maternal care, infant and preschool health, handicapped child services, school health, communicable disease control, mental health, mobile meals, and health maintenance centers. The agency's staff is located in five locations, decentralized throughout the service area, each with a generalized home visit caseload.

In 1970 the VNA staff began to make changes in the clinical record and computer system. While the changes began independently, their inter-dependence soon became apparent, as did the lack of a standard client classification of health or health-related problems. This lack not only hindered the documentation of nursing services, but also the development of specific nursing interventions, communication among health disciplines, and nursing research efforts.

A project to develop a classification of client problems addressed by nurses in a community health setting was begun under a contract negotiated between the VNA of Omaha and the Division of Nursing, DHEW. Part of the project was the development of a manual: *A Classification Scheme for Client Problems in Community Health Nursing*, now in its third printing.

The project began with a pilot study using 338 families newly admitted to care. Each nurse assessed the family unit and the individual members utilizing a defined data base.

In order to facilitate sorting all the data generated by the pilot study, it was necessary to differentiate between nursing and non-nursing problems, individual health and family health problems; and actual and potential problems. The nursing problems categorization included risk factors, etiology, and lab tests so they were referred to as descriptors rather than signs or symptoms. Using an inductive approach, like descriptors were grouped and a uniform name for each problem was developed.

The classroom consisted of four categories of problems. This classification was then tested. Using the pilot study's classification scheme, nurses listed each nursing problem. All nurses were encouraged to add or delete problem names and descriptors; and these changes were incorporated into the classification. The result consisted of a scheme with four categories, 49 problems and descriptors for each problem.

By 1976, the staff of the VNA of Omaha began using the classification system in all their home visit clinical records. It was understood that the classification scheme needed further refinement, yet use in the clinical setting was necessary to establish validity and elicit feedback from actual practitioners.

The VNA project was extended by a second contract to field test the classification in other community health agencies. In addition, the project included development of a manual, completing statistical analysis of comparative data among the test agencies, and beginning an expected outcomes and outcome criteria component. The field tests involved a combination agency, an official agency, and a voluntary agency. These were the Des Moines Public Health Nursing Association; the State of Delaware Department of Health and Social Services, Division of Public Health; and the Dallas VNA. Representatives from the three agencies participated in developing the test methodology.

Using the data base and the classification scheme, the field-test nurse listed problem labels and significant descriptors, and submitted a copy of the initial assessment and the problem list. The problem list of the test agency was compared to that of the project staff. New labels and desciptors for the 49 problems, as well as differences in usage among testers, were incorporated. The refinement of the problem classification scheme resulted in 38 problems and four areas or domains in which nursing interventions occur:

Environmental: The material resources and physical surroundings of the home, neighborhood, and broader community.

Psychosocial: Patterns of behavior, communications, relationships, and development.

Physiological: The functional status of the processes that maintain life.

Health Behaviors: Activities that maintain or produce wellness; promote recovery; or maximize rehabilitation.

The descriptors were refined to include only signs and symptoms. Those signs and symptoms are almost mutually exclusive. An example of a problem with a cluster of signs and symptoms follows:

Environmental Domain
03. *Safety hazards* (:)
    A. (:) *Residence*
        01. structurally unsound
        02. inadequate heat
        03. steep stairs
        04. obstructed exits/entries
        05. cluttered living space
        06. unsafe storage of dangerous objects/substances
        07. unsafe mats and throw rugs
        08. locks needed safety devices
        09. iead base paint present
        10. unsafe gas/electrical appliances
        11. other
    B. (:) *Neighborhood*
        01. high crime rate
        02. high pollution level (e.g., noise, air, waste)

03. uncontrolled animals
04. high traffic area
05. other

"Other" appears as the last entry in every sign/symptom cluster indicating that the cluster is open-ended, allowing the nurse to write in a sign or or symptom.

For the expected outcomes and outcome criteria of the project—definitions, rationale, and data collection was also planned. Data collection tools or forms were completed by all the Omaha staff nurses. They established a data base, nursing problem list using the problem classification scheme, and appropriate expected outcomes and outcome criteria. The next goal was to produce and pilot-test expected outcome/outcome criterion schemes that conformed to the problem classification scheme.

Preparing to make a home visit, the community health nurse asks, "What will happen?" and "When will it happen?" An expected outcome is the statement of an intended or realistically anticipated change, improvement, or solution of a nursing problem at a specified point in time as a result of nursing intervention; and it is usually synonymous with general client objective, goal, nursing prognosis, standard for evaluation, and terminal expectation.

Outcome criterion is defined as a statement that increases the specificity and measurement potential of the expected outcome by describing how a client will look, feel, or behave at a specified point in time as a result of nursing intervention. This is usually synonymous with specific client objective, goal indicator, behavioral criterion, and action appraisal. The questions are now "How will I know?" "How will the client look, feel, and behave?" Conceptualization of the family nursing process served as the necessary bridge, linking this project with the literature, the problem classification scheme, and with future research anticipated by our agency, and the actual nursing practice of our staff.

The revised and refined problem classification scheme was used to develop a problem list for each record. After data assessment and analysis were completed, expected outcome and outcome criteria were revised and refined.

Forty staff nurses from the Omaha, Dallas, Des Moines, and Delaware agencies, randomly selected, participated in the testing. The three agency representatives from Dallas, Des Moines, and Delaware came to Omaha to receive instructions and materials to take home and present to their own staff.

Data resulting from the field test were again analyzed using three methods: percent of agreement, Kendall's coefficient of concordance, and Spearmen rank correlation coefficient. A posttest was conducted to assess reliability of the schemes over a period of time. As before, the expected outcome/outcome criteria schemes were revised and refined based on testing data. In 1980, the schemes were implemented in the VNA to determine their value in the real world; establishing validity and eliciting feedback from actual practitioners.

The current expected outcome and outcome criteria schemes are designed to reflect reasonable, measurable client behaviors that can be observed and monitored by the community health nurse. The goals are not to prevent that nurse from thinking, but rather to encourage thought and to measure the measurable, not the immeasurable. The terms prevention, improvement, and maintenance, are expected outcome choices: our data collection produced 580 expected outcome statements. These reduced to three expectd outcomes capable of application to all 38 problems in the problem classification scheme.

Outcome criteria statements developed during data collection were also tested and modified. The original 2,125 statements were revised, refined, and ordered into 202 statements and then into 188 statements. These 188 statements were organized into clusters. Unlike the expected outcomes that are applicable to all problem labels, an outcome criterion cluster appears for each problem of the problem classification scheme. An example follows:

Safety hazards (:)

    A. (:) Residence
- a. Identifies/selected plans to reduce safety hazards (e.g., focuses on specific problems, considers options, sets priorities)
- b. Uses assistive/protective measures (e.g., grab bar, rail, lock, non-skid strip, smoke alarm, gate/screen, decal, persons)
- c. Removes obstructions from floors/hallways (e.g., clutter, loose carpet, sharp objects)
- d. Installs/repairs housing essentials (e.g., furnishings, appliances, heat, cool, plumbing, lighting, storage, structure)
- e. Reports/demonstrates no accidents/injuries (e.g., due to falls, burns, pests, poisons)
- f. Uses resources for search/move to other housing (e.g., self, relatives, friends, community agencies)
- g. Other

    B. (:) Neighborhood
- a. Identifies/selects plans to reduce safety hazards (e.g., focuses on specific problems, considers options, sets priorities)
- b. Installs/uses protective devices (e.g., lock, light, alarms, fence)
- c. Communicates/cooperates with neighbors (e.g., care of property/children/pets)
- d. Uses resources for search/move to other housing (e.g., self, relatives, friends, community agencies)
- e. Other

The initial goal of the VNA project was to improve delivery, documentation, and description of client care. Since potential for computerization was recognized early, the agency was able to modify hardware and develop software. Thus the VNA of Omaha was able to improve orientation and assimilation of new nursing staff. The staff was able to enhance family assessment and planning; they were better able to sort and organize pertinent data which leads to nursing intervention. There was an increased efficiency and effectiveness in the recording procedure. With standard nomenclature, improved communication between staff nurses and between the staff and supervisors occurred. Also, better agencywide program planning was created through the use of client and management information systems.

And, finally, acceptable documentation for third-party payers, professional auditors, and utilization review committee members followed using nursing diagnoses as a basis for reimbursing nursing service. Thus, this extended project provided community health nurses with tools—not burdens—capable of improving service to their clients and their own nursing practice.

ABOUT THE AUTHOR

At the time of writing, Karen Martin, MSN, RN, was responsible for conducting a research contract with the Division of Nursing, U.S. Department of Health and Human Services, and for the staff development program of the Visiting Nurses Association of Omaha, Omaha, Nebraska.

REFERENCES

1. *A Classification Scheme for Client Problems in Community Health Nursing*, DHHS Pub. No. (HRA) 80-16. Available from National Technical Information Service, Springfield, VA.

Evaluating Patient Outcomes

Frances Inzer and Mary Jo Aspinall

Most community health nurses have by now incorporated goal statements into documentation. However, appropriate evaluation of progress— comparing the patient outcome to the specified goals—remains a recurrent dilemma in community health. "Goals met" is no longer considered an adequate statement for patient evaluation, this 1981 article is reprinted in full as an excellent example of scaling (quantifying) goal attainment. Recognizing that without specificity, recordings are unreliable as indicators of patient progress, the authors describe a system to evaluate nonnumerical goals in which nurses independently identify components of a goal and develop a scale to measure its achievement. Although originally developed in a hospital setting, the concepts may be readily applied to the community health practice setting.

Every nurse who has ever developed a care plan knows the importance of formulating patient goals. In the past, nursing activities were often included in these goals; however, in recent years nurses have developed goal statements in terms of patient outcome behavior. The word "outcome" is generally accepted to mean the end result of an activity, rather than the activity itself. Examples of goal statements for patient outcome behavior are: "will be free of chest pain,"

Reprinted with permission from *Nursing Outlook*, 29 (March 1981), copyright © 1981, American Journal of Nursing Company, pp. 178-181.

"will ambulate the length of the hall," and "will demonstrate colostomy care." These goals indicate a focus on the patient's end behavior, not the nurse's action.

Currently, considerable attention is being given to the development of outcome criteria as a measurement tool in the evaluation process. Such criteria are being utilized in quality assurance programs, nursing audits, standards for accreditation of hospitals, and standards for nursing practice. For instance, Standard IV of the American Nurses' Association's *Standards for Medical-Surgical Nursing Practice* stipulates that in evaluation of the nursing care plan, "patient response is compared with observable outcomes which are specified in the goals."[1]

OBJECTIVE MEASUREMENTS

As with all new concepts, however, the ideas are intellectually adopted before they are actually put into practice. In reviewing a number of patient (medical) records, we found that most nurses record patient responses in judgmental, interpretive terms—such as "seems to be more comfortable," "wound appears to be healing"—instead of in specific behavioral terminology. Upon closer examination, the identification of specific criteria that could be used as an index for evaluation by all nurses who recorded the patient's response was strikingly absent. For example, one nurse may have recorded that the patient was increasing in ambulation when he could walk from the bed to the chair, whereas another nurse may have stated he achieved this goal when he could walk the length of the corridor. Without specificity, recordings are unreliable as indicators of patient progress.

In searching the literature, a number of articles identified the need to refine objective methods of measuring patient progress as basic to building the science of nursing. For the most part, however, there are relatively few articles describing tools that operationalize evaluation of goal attainment. In one article, Zimmer and others describe prototype sets of health outcome criteria that they developed for specific patient populations.[2] They defined increment measurements for each criterion and demonstrated how each could be scaled for measurement purposes.

Since there has been limited scientific testing of scales to measure patient progress, we raised the question: Is it feasible to utilize observable patient behavioral data to develop a practical, incremental scale for measuring patient outcome behavior in relation to goal attainment? The answer to this question came, in part, from a study in which a group of RNs on three surgical wards at the Veterans Administration Medical Center, Long Beach, California, participated. The study, reported by Hefferin, evaluated the effectiveness of experimental treatment by the degree and rate of the patient's goal attainment.[3]

FORMULATING GOALS

Prior to the study period, patient goals which were recorded on nursing care plans in the study wards were surveyed in order to determine the type of goals that would require scaling. Since many goals were stated in general, nonspecific terms such as "will be able to care for self after discharge," "will return to board and care home," it was apparent that nurses would first need help in learning to state goals in specific, measurable terms.

Once they had mastered formulating goal statements, the next task was developing scales to measure the attainment of the goals. A modified version of the standard Goal Attainment Scaling (GAS) method, described by Kiresuk, was utilized.[4] This method calls for a goal-continuum of five relatively equal increments for each goal. For the study, the patient's initial status was made. Step 1. Four other steps or levels, depicting progressive goal achievement, were then developed with Step 5 indicating goal attainment. Through this five-point scale, measurement of the patient's progress toward the goal could be made at specified time intervals.

DEVELOPING SCALES

Goals involving a numerical component were fairly easy to scale, while other goals were more difficult because of their abstract nature. Examples of goals with a numerical component are: "to lose 10 pounds," "to reduce the blood pressure by 10 mm Hg." Scaling a numerical goal is illustrated in Example 1 (see Fig. 1).

After this relatively easy task, we directed our attention to finding a system to evaluate non-numerical goals such as "to care for colostomy without assistance." However, in reaching this goal, several activities are involved—that is, removing the bag, irrigating the colon, cleansing the stoma, and applying a new bag. Mindful of the old adage about mixing apples and oranges, it was decided to experiment with a separate subgoal for each component and use a scale to measure attainment for each. Example 2 illustrates one subgoal attainment scale.

This method of scaling subgoals did not seem to be a feasible solution, however, because it was difficult to gauge what 25 percent, 50 percent, etc., would be. Another problem was how to measure the patient's total ability to accomplish all the subgoals without assistance, since a patient could be at Step 2 of one subgoal and Step 5 of another at the same point in time.

We then tried another approach to scale the main goal by incorporating attainment of each subgoal in a progressive manner as shown in Example 3. But, we quickly recognized the problems with this method; some patients did not progress in the order in which elements of the steps were written. For instance, some patients could apply a new bag without assistance, but they could not remove the soiled bag without assistance.

FIGURE 1
Examples of Goal Attainment Scaling

Example 1. *Goal: To lose 10 pounds of weight*

Step 1	Step 2	Step 3	Step 4	Step 5
Weighs 190 pounds (present weight)	Weighs 187-189 pounds	Weighs 184-186 pounds	Weighs 181-183 pounds	Weighs 180 pounds or less (desired weight)

Example 2. *Goal: To care for colostomy without assistance*
Subgoal: To remove soiled bag

Step 1	Step 2	Step 3	Step 4	Step 5
Can not do task without assistance	Can do 25% of task without assistance	Can do 50% of task without assistance	Can do 75% of task without assistance	Can do 100% of task without assistance

Example 3. *Goal: To care for colostomy without assistance*

Step 1	Step 2	Step 3	Step 4	Step 5
Unable to do any care without assistance	Able to remove soiled bag without assistance	Able to remove soiled bag and irrigate without assistance	Able to remove soiled bag, irrigate, and cleanse stoma without assistance	Able to remove soiled bag, irrigate cleanse stoma, and apply new bag without assistance

Example 4. *Goal: To care for colostomy without assistance*
Four components: Remove soiled bag—irrigate—cleanse stoma—apply new bag

Step 1	Step 2	Step 3	Step 4	Step 5
Does none of above without assistance	Does one of above without assistance	Does two of above without assistance	Does three of above without assistance	Does four of above without assistance

The format that was finally adopted listed all components of the goal. Each step indicated the number of components the patient could perform, regardless of the sequence in which the patient accomplished the task (see Example 4). This method seemed to differentiate effectively between levels of goal achievement and was easily understandable to the nurses.

USING PATIENT OUTCOMES SCALES

A few of the nurses, after seeing one example of this method, could independently identify components of a goal and develop a scale to measure its achievement. Others had difficulty in analyzing activities that a patient had to complete to achieve a goal. The problems ranged from those nurses who could not identify any integral activities to those who identified too many activities, most of which did not pertain to the goal.

Obviously, many of the nurses needed to develop skills in both analyzing patient goals and synthesizing essential elements or activities into the goal. We used a directed thought process during the training period to help them achieve these skills, that is, we asked the following questions:

> Tell me what a patient will have to do in order to walk on crutches. Will he be able to get out of bed alone? Does he need to learn how to move himself to the side of the bed? Are quad set exercises essential to his walking? What is the outcome you expect of the patient as a result of your using the Nelson bed? If he needs to climb stairs as well as walk on level surfaces, then shouldn't the goal be stated 'to walk with crutches on level surfaces and stairs'?

With guided practice, all of the nurses developed the ability to analyze a goal and divide it into component parts, which were stated as patient outcomes rather than nursing actions. They also learned to synthesize essential elements into a comprehensive goal when certain activities were not included in the original goal statement. The complexity of this task is shown in Example 5 (see Fig. 2), which was written for a patient with right total hip prosthesis.

We were concerned that the nurses would tend to use the same scale, perhaps inappropriately, for another patient with the same goal. Although some duplication occurred, the nurses individualized the scale if different component activities were involved. For example, a patient with a Symes procedure needs to learn to walk with crutches as does a patient with a total hip prosthesis. However, since most patients with a Symes procedure have no problem with quad sets and straight leg raising, this is not an appropriate activity for them. Instead, they need to learn balancing, since they cannot toe touch. The goal for a patient with this condition is scaled in Example 6.

FIGURE 2
Examples of Goal Attainment Scaling

Example 5. *Goal: To walk with crutches (right leg toe touching only) on level surfaces and stairs*

Four components: Do 10 consecutive quad sets and 10 consecutive straight leg raises— transfer from bed to chair (or guerney) —walk with parallel bars with right leg toe touching—walk with crutches on stairs

Step 1	Step 2	Step 3	Step 4	Step 5
Does none of above	Does one of above	Does two of above	Does three of above	Does four of above

Example 6. *Goal: To walk with crutches (patient with 2nd stage Symes, left foot)*

Seven components: Transfer from bed to chair by self—rise from chair and stand—balance on right foot without support —stand on toes of right foot while holding to chair—hop on one foot while holding to a stationary chair —hop on one foot while moving along parallel bars—walk with crutches

Step 1	Step 2	Step 3	Step 4	Step 5
Does none of above	Does one or two of above	Does three or four of above	Does five or six of above	Does all of above

Another demonstration of individualizing a scale is shown in Examples 7 and 8 (see Fig. 3). These two scales evaluate range of motion of the upper extremity for patients with different surgical conditions. Although only one goal was needed to assess progress in a few patients in the study, most patients were evaluated in attaining two or three goals. For instance, a patient with an amputation might have a goal for stump healing for prosthesis fit in addition to the goal of walking with crutches. In this situation, both Example 5 and Example 9 goals would be evaluated for this patient.

In using the scales, it became obvious that a five-point scale was easier with four components or multiples of four. Many nurses had a tendency to list four components, omitting a fifth if it did not seem too vital. This practice did not seem to be a disadvantage, since components usually were carefully weighed to select the most essential. We consistently used a five-point scale because the data were being statistically evaluated in a research project. However, any combination of intervals of four, six, or other numbered scales could be used in most practice settings.

Most of the examples cited are discharge goals, which are usually appropriate for most surgical patients because of the short length of their hospitalization. For a few patients who had complications, a longer stay in the hospital was required. In these instances, the nurses had to learn to write more basic goals because these patients progressed more slowly. For example, ambulating without assistance would require a considerable period of time for a 78-year-old male, weighing 200 pounds, who had a resection of an abdominal aortic aneurysm. One goal for this patient is stated in Example 10.

SUMMARY

In this study, nurses effectively demonstrated that in addition to stating goals in observable outcomes, they could develop rating scales to measure a patient's progress toward goal attainment. An unexpected finding was that improvement in evaluation was accompanied by corresponding improvement in other components of the nursing process. For example, prior to the study period, nurses rarely listened to chest sounds or measured ventilatory volume to assess lung congestion, even though many had received training in physical assessment and a respirometer was available on the unit. During the study period, however, there was a flurry of auscultation and spirometric measurement activities for patients whose goals were to decrease lung congestion. When one such patient failed to progress as rapidly as the nurse anticipated, greater assistance was given to pulmonary physiotherapy and assistance with coughing.

Although nursing has not given sufficient attention to the development of patient evaluation tools, recent legislation as well as consumers' demand for quality care are providing the impetus for developing such mechanisms

FIGURE 3
Examples of Goal Attainment Scaling

Example 7. *Goal: To increase the range of motion of the left shoulder (patient with left transcervical fracture)*
Four components: Can extend left upper extremity forward—can extend left upper extremity sideways
—Can do circular motion of left upper extremity—can raise and lower shoulders

Step 1	Step 2	Step 3	Step 4	Step 5
Does none of above	Does one of above	Does two of above	Does three of above	Does four of above

Example 8. *Goal: To increase range of motion of right arm (patient with thoracotomy and right lower lobe lobectomy)*
Four components: Can raise arm straight in front—can raise arm straight to side
—can raise arm straight overhead—can raise arm and reach to back

Step 1	Step 2	Step 3	Step 4	Step 5
Does none of above	Does one of above	Does two of above	Does three of above	Does four of above

Example 9. *Goal: To have a healed stump*
Four components: No swelling—no drainage—no pain or exceptionally tender spots—presence of granulation tissue

Step 1	Step 2	Step 3	Step 4	Step 5
Has none of above	Has one of above	Has two of above	Has three of above	Has four of above

Example 10. *Goal: To get out of bed without assistance*
Four components: Move to side of bed without assistance—swing both legs over side of bed without assistance
—get to a sitting position on the side of bed without assistance—push self up to a standing position

Step 1	Step 2	Step 3	Step 4	Step 5
Does none of above	Does one of above	Does two of above	Does three of above	Does four of above

in a scientific way. This fact may significantly contribute to refining clinical data for the objective evaluation of patient progress. Since most nurses receive some theoretical education in the evaluation process, the challenge may well be to provide nurses, in both educational and service settings, with practical experiences in developing and implementing evaluation techniques.

REFERENCES

1. *Standards of Medical-Surgical Nursing Practice,* (Kansas City, MO: American Nurses' Association, 1974).

2. M. J. Zimmer, et al., *Development of Sets of Patient Health Outcome Criteria by Panels of Nurse Experts,* Final Report of Project No. 7 (Madison: Wisconsin Regional Medical Program, University of Wisconsin Hospitals Nursing Service, and University of Wisconsin-Milwaukee School of Nursing, 1974).

3. Elizabeth Hefferin, "Health Goal Setting: Patient-Nurse Collaboration at Veterans Administration Facilities," *Military Medicine,* 144 (December 1979), 814-822.

4. T. J. Kiresuk and R. E. Sherman, "Goal Attainment Scaling: A General Method for Evaluating Comprehensive Mental Health Programs," *Community Mental Health Journal,* (December 1968), 443-453.

Home Health Nursing Care Plans

E. Joyce Gould and Joan Wargo

Creating nursing goal statements that realistically indicate the behavior expected from patients or significant others is becoming more complex with early discharges of acutely ill patients, a shortage of adequately prepared community health nurses, and tightening standards for reimbursement. This recently published edition of Home Health Nursing Care Plans *provides a guide to assist the home care nurse in developing care plans that identify and solve complex nursing diagnoses. In addition to excerpts from the introduction and the guide to using the standardized care plans, we have reprinted here one example of a nursing care plan from this manual.*

INTRODUCTION

This is the era of constricting Medicare reimbursement, demands for more documentation, increased litigation against health care organizations and individual professionals, and demands by consumers and third-party payers to assure the quality of health care provided. Furthermore, the home care nurse is challenged to provide care for patients with increasingly complex illnesses at the same time that there are more demands for a written description of care provided to the patient.

In a medicare-certified home health agency, the nurse's primary responsibilities include working to enable patients to become independent of the home care agency by teaching them and their caregivers the skills necessary to manage their health needs. Nursing strategies must incorporate methods to assure that patients receive effective care and to measure whether patients meet treatment goals. For home care, patient teaching is one of the key nursing interventions. However, documentation of patient education has often been cursory because of time constraints.

Given this environment of increased demands, the administrative and clinical staff at United Home Health Services sought to devise a charting system that would facilitate documentation, meet professional standards, follow legal guidelines, justify third-party payment, and define quality of care in terms of patient outcomes. In our experience, these nursing care plans fulfill these needs. Time spent writing the nursing narrative note is greatly reduced. Patient education is systematized and a consistent approach to patient teaching is encouraged even when teaching is performed by different nurses. Progress toward meeting preset goals is reviewed automatically at each visit.

New nurses find the care plans invaluable in identifying and solving complex multiple nursing diagnoses. These plans also assist in the orientation of staff and students who are new to the practice of home health nursing. Coordination of appropriate therapies necessary for patient care is included as part of the nursing orders. These care plans define standards of nursing care for the quality assurance program. The format of the care plans facilitates thorough documentation required by third party payers. Much of the charting can be completed during the home visit.

The care plans include those nursing diagnoses that originate from medical problems, as well as those that address special clinical management situations. There is a section of care plans pertaining to the needs of patients receiving intravenous, parenteral, and enteral therapies.

Many of the diagnoses included here have been accepted for clinical testing by the North American Nursing Diagnosis Association. Because diagnostic categories are the result of an evolving process, nursing practice is broader and more complex than the currently accepted complement of diagnoses. At this stage of diagnostic development, the decision was made to design additional nursing diagnoses to address issues relevant to the clinical practice of home care nurses in a medicare-certified home health agency.

The standardized nursing care plans included in this book are the result of more than three years of development by the staff of United Home Health Services. They are offered as a usable tool or a starting point for further refinement and adaptation by other home care nurses.

PATIENT-CENTERED GOALS

To be patient centered, a goal must indicate what behavior is expected from the patient or significant other as a result of nursing intervention. Realistic goals must be stated as precisely as possible. Each goal should focus on one behavior that is directly observable or assessable. However, a goal does *not* describe what the nurse does. Rather the goal should describe what will be done, whether the patient or significant other will do it, when it will be accomplished, and what standard of performance is expected.

Taking time to work with the patient and family to decide which goals to work toward is critical to success. Establishing achievable goals is the heart of the nursing care plan, because they give direction and guidance to nursing care and serve as criteria to evaluate the results of care. In addition, they function as a common language among the nursing staff and thus enhance the continuity of patient care.

Statements of goals can refer to overt or covert behavior. *Recite, list, sort* and *demonstrate* are verbs that indicate overt performances. *Recognize, comprehend, judge,* and *know* are verbs that reflect the utilization of mental or cognitive processes, i.e., covert performances. Another way to classify behaviors is to divide them into three domains: psychomotor, affective, and cognitive.[1] The psychomotor domain includes motor skills referred to by such verbs as *administer, demonstrate, practice, show,* and *assist.* The affective domain covers expression of feelings, interests, attitudes, and values that are referred to by performance verbs such as *listen, touch, ignore, regard,* and *share.* The cognitive domain deals with intellectual abilities referred to by such verbs as *explore, inform, discuss, list,* and *evaluate.*

The following questions can be used as a checklist to determine if the goal is realistic and measurable.

Does the statement of the *goal:*

- have only one performance verb?
- indicate an achievable performance?
- identify an activity which is directly observable or assessable?
- describe what will be done by the patient and/or significant other?
- state when the goal will be accomplished?
- indicate the standard of performance?

USING STANDARDIZED NURSING CARE PLANS

The care plans in this book can be used in a number of ways to assist the home care nurse in providing and documenting nursing care.

1. *Clinical Record.* Nursing care plans can be copied and inserted

into a patient's chart to guide the delivery of nursing care and to document the process and outcome of care given.

2. *Patient Education System.* The teaching plan portion of each care plan is an outline of what the patient or significant other must learn in order to manage the health problem(s).

3. *Quality Assurance Standards.* Each nursing care plan sets the standards of care and the outcomes expected as a result of nursing care. The nursing orders could be used in a process audit to review any agency's own charting system to determine the appropriateness of nursing care provided. The contributing objectives could be used to determine, from any agency's clinical record, if a patient has met the learning objectives.

4. *Charting Guide.* Nursing staff and students can review a specific nursing care plan to determine the relevant items that should be documented in any clinical record.

5. *Reference Book.* This book can be used as a reference to assist nursing staff with writing their own nursing plans.

6. *Orientation Manual.* New staff can consult the nursing orders and teaching plans to determine what care should be provided during a home visit for each nursing diagnosis.

7. *Utilization Review.* Establishing goal dates when care is initiated encourages nurse and patient to work toward timely discharge. The accomplishment of learning objectives indicates discharge is approaching. Agency standards can be developed regarding the number of visits expected for each care plan.

8. *Discharge Assessment of Hospitalized Patients..* Use the teaching plan as an assessment tool to determine whether the patient has accomplished each objective. If not, patient may require referral to home care agency for follow-up.

9. *Textbook.* Nursing students in undergraduate programs can use this book in planning, delivering, and documenting patient care.

10. *Justify Reimbursement.* Documentation on these care plans can provide a more complete description of the patient teaching provided. It also indicates the specific knowledge deficits that require nursing intervention.

11. *Litigation Risk Management.* Thorough documentation of patient education and what the patient or significant other learned as a result of the instruction given is a significant step toward reducing the likelihood of a successful lawsuit against the agency or the nurse. These completed care plans can assist in developing a successful defense when a patient claims he was harmed in carrying out self-care activities during the provision of agency services or after discharge.

FIGURE 1
Example of Nursing Care Plan

Nursing Care Plan for _____ Adm. # _____ Date _____
Nursing Diagnosis: Impaired skin integrity of lower extremity related to vascular insufficiency, resulting
      in **necrotic lesion(s)**
Goal: Patient/significant other will understand treatment modality necessary to restore skin integrity and
      prevent infection.

NURSING ORDERS

1. Assess involved area (edema, temperature, color, peripheral pulses, sensation).
2. Assess other extremity.
3. Assess and document character of lesion(s).
4. Encourage medication compliance.
5. Advise patient/significant other in methods to promote effective circulation.
6. Alert physician to change in status.
7. Evaluate safety in transfers and ability to use assistive devices.
8. Evaluate personal care needs and arrange appropriate intervention.
9. Instruct in disease process.
10. Arrange for and/or provide necessary medical supplies.
11. Provide patient education materials: _____.

_____

Nurse's Signature _____

TEACHING PLAN

Contributing Objectives	Dates Instructed												Goal Date
Patient/S.O. Will													Date Accom.
Identify signs of increased vascular and tissue involvement.													
Demonstrate the ability to perform prescribed treatment.													
Participate in personal care needs.													
Demonstrate safe transfers and use of assistive devices.													
Demonstrate an understanding of disease process and risk factors (PVD = impaired peripheral blood flow, varicose veins or dilated veins with incompetent valves).													

Joan Wargo, RN, BSN

FIG. 1 (continued)

Nursing Care Plan for _____ Adm. #_____

Contributing Objectives	Dates Instructed															Goal Date / Date Accom.
Patient/S.O. Will																
List measures to promote effective circulation: (a) ankle-pumping, (b) elevation, (c) avoidance of constrictive clothing (garters, knee-highs).																
Accept and listen to instruction concerning patient education materials.																
Identify symptoms requiring medical intervention.																
INITIALS																

KEY

I = Instruction   E = Evaluation   N = Narrative   C = Care Given   D = Discussion   S = Supervision

Initials	Signature	Title

ABOUT THE AUTHORS

E. Joyce Gould, MSN, RN, is Assistant Administrator for Clinical Services, United Home Health Services, Philadelphia, Pennsylvania, and at the University of Pennsylvania, Philadelphia. Joan Wargo, BSN, RN, C, is a primary nurse, United Home Health Services.

REFERENCES

1. Barbara Klug Redman. *The Process of Patient Teaching in Nursing Practice;* 5th ed. (St. Louis: C. V. Mosby, 1984).

Guide for the Development
of the Nursing Care Plan

Visiting Nurse Association of Metropolitan Detroit

*Client outcome statements with specific time frames are a necessary com-
ponent of community health nursing program objectives. The Visiting Nurse
Association of Metropolitan Detroit's* Guide for the Development of the
Nursing Care Plan *provides another tool to assist nurses in writing a care
plan that realistically describes the intended outcome of nursing care with
a specified time frame for achieving nursing goals.*

*The newly revised introduction to the manual, written by Charlene
Cotting, MSN, RN, District Director of the Visiting Nurse Association of
Metropolitan Detroit, describes the use of the expected outcome statements
and criteria and introduces the examples presented here of the formats
developed by the Detroit VNA.*

INTRODUCTION

The Visiting Nurse Association of Metropolitan Detroit has developed expected
outcome statements and criteria for each of the nursing diagnoses it uses. These
nursing diagnoses are based on the taxonomy developed by the Third Conference on
Nursing Diagnosis. Nursing management protocols were also developed for each
diagnosis. (An example of a nursing management protocol is shown in Figure 1.)

FIGURE 1
Example of Nursing Management Protocol

Nursing Diagnoses and Management Protocols

Impairment of Skin/Mucosa/Tissues Integrity Related to _____

I. Defining Characteristics

Disruption of skin/mucosal/tissue surfaces

Destruction of skin/mucosal/tissue layers

Invasion of body structure

Alteration in color

Alteration in temperature

Alteration in sensation

Alteration in turgor

Alteration in secretions

Alteration in pigmentation

Alteration in contour

Alteration in density

Alteration in humidity of the skin/mucosal tissue/tissue surfaces

Presence of mechanical forces

Presence of immobility

Presence of irritants to the skin/mucosa/tissue

II. Nursing Interventions

Nursing Treatments

Reduce and/or remove causes of impaired skin/mucosa/tissue integrity (e.g., immobility, altered nutritional state, mechanical irritants)

Frequent and proper position changes

Good skin care with attention to skin over bony prominences (discourage excessive use of soaps which are high in alkali)

Dry, clean, wrinkle-free bed linen

Use of sheepskin pads for bony prominences; soft, protective pads for heels and elbows, and alternating air pressure mattress

Refrain from local cold applications

Expose affected areas to air

Activity program as ordered (e.g., active/passive range of motion to increase skin and vascular tone)

Good oral hygiene

Massage area as indicated to increase circulation

Maintain comfortable room temperature with adequate humidification

Refrain from simultaneously powdering and lubricating skin

Use paper or transparent tape instead of adhesive tape

Pain control measures (e.g., position changes, medication, diversional activities, massage)

Implement medical regimen, including prescribed treatment program for existing wound problem (e.g., Karaya procedure, cleansing with hydogen peroxide, PhisoDerm or antibiotic solution, application of antacids, corticosteroids, oxygen under pressure, and heat)

Safe disposal of soiled dressings

Consult with appropriate professional staff

Provide emotional support

Nursing Observations

Monitor vital signs (increased temperature, tachycardia with infectious process)

Response to treatment program (e.g., changes in color, size, depth, and drainage—serous fluid, pus, or blood)

Health Teaching

Explain causes of impaired skin/mucosa/tissue integrity

Rationale and intended effect of treatment program

Signs and symptoms of altered skin/mucosa/tissue integrity designating those to be reported

Principles of good nutrition and composition of well-balanced meals (increased calories, increased protein as indicated)

Administration of medications and side effects

Use of equipment and safety precautions (e.g., air pressure mattress, circoelectric bed, flotation pad, whirlpool bath)

Nursing treatments as appropriate

Since health problems differ in severity and chronicity among patients, three different levels of outcome statements have been written for each nursing diagnosis. The outcome levels are based on a conceptual framework adapted from the Karnosky Performance Status Scale and the "Levels of Applications of Preventive Measures" by Leavell and Clark (see Fig. 2).

The expected outcome statements for each nursing diagnosis are developed to address three discrete areas: (a) the patient, family, or caregiver's knowledge of the health problem (i.e., nursing diagnosis); (b) skills or resources necessary to resolve, improve, or manage the health problem; and (c) patient status related to the health problem. These three areas are addressed separately because it cannot be assumed that a positive outcome in one area guarantees a positive outcome in other areas. For example, being knowledgeable about the signs and symptoms, complications, and influencing factors of the nursing diagnosis does not necessarily guarantee that the patient or family will be willing or able to make the appropriate behavioral and life-style changes necessary to adhere to the prescribed treatment plan. Nor does adherence to the prescribed treatment plan guarantee the desired impact on the actual health problem. Stating expected outcomes for each of these three areas also helps to more clearly document the "skilled care" components of service and to more clearly communicate the patient's progress. Thus, the patient may have achieved one or two of the expected outcomes, but not the third. In this case, the achieved outcomes would no longer be considered a problem. Only the unachieved outcome would be addressed on subsequent visits. The nurse, in writing a care plan, must choose the level that most reasonably and realistically describes the intended outcome of VNA service for each nursing diagnosis.

There are two components to each expected outcome. The first is the outcome statement. The outcome statement is a measurable statement of the behavior of the patient, family, or caregiver that is expected to be achieved as a result of the care provided. Examples of outcome statement are:

- The patient demonstrates knowledge related to alteration in respiratory status.
- The patient demonstrates measures to control decreased cardiac output.
- The patient achieves a stable respiratory status.

The second component of each expected outcome is the outcome criteria. Outcome criteria are actions or behaviors that are necessary to the achievement of the outcome statement. For example, if the patient is able to verbalize the signs and symptoms, influencing factors, and complications of decreased caridac output, then he or she has achieved the expected outcome that the patient demonstrate knowledge related to decreased cardiac output.

For each level of the expected outcomes there are three outcome statements and appropriate criteria (see example in Fig.3). In writing the nursing care plan,

FIGURE 2
Nursing Diagnoses Levels with Associated Outcome Foci and Nursing Interventions

Levels of Nursing Diagnosis and Characteristics of Altered Health Status	Outcome Focus	Nursing Interventions[*]
Level I • "At risk" populations • Minor interruptions in life activities • Able to continue normal activities with minimal effort and/or assistance • Minor signs/symptoms of altered health status	• Prevent/correct altered health status • Prevent complications/sequelae of altered health status • Prevent/minimize disability • Achieve/maintain normal functioning	Interventions include: • Direct physical care • Teaching • Monitoring • Emotional support • Coordination of services • Referral • Assistance in home adaptation
Level II • Unable to carry on normal activity • Unable to live at home but requires varying amounts of assistance • Progressive signs/symptoms of altered health status • Presence of minor complications/sequelae of altered health status	• Correct/control/improve altered health status • Prevent further complications/sequelae • Achieve normal/improved functioning • Prevent/minimize prolonged disability	Interventions include: • Direct physical care • Teaching • Monitoring • Emotional support • Coordination of services • Referral • Assistance in home adaptation
Level III • Unable to care for self • Requires total or nearly total assistance • Without strong caregiver support, consider institutionalization • Advanced signs/symptoms of altered health status • Presence of complications/sequelae of altered health status	• Control/improve/manage altered health status • Control complications/sequelae of altered health status • Restoration of the individual to optimal level of functioning within constraints of disability	Interventions include: • Direct physical care • Teaching • Monitoring • Emotional support • Coordination of services • Referral • Assistance in home adaptation

* Interventions vary with severity of altered health status and availability of support systems.

Adapted from: Karnofsky Performance Status Scale and E. G. Clark, and H. R. Leavell *Preventive Medicine for the Doctor in His Community* (3d ed.; New York: McGraw-Hill Book Co., 1965), p. 20.

the outcome statement is used as written and the outcome criteria are translated into nursing actions (see Figs. 4 and 5).

In most instances, all three expected outcomes will be necessary for each nursing diagnosis. However, if the assessment data indicate that one or more of the expected outcomes have already been met, then it/they need not be included in the care plan.

GUIDELINES FOR USE OF THE EXPECTED OUTCOME STATEMENTS AND CRITERIA

1. All three expected outcome statements are necessary for each nursing diagnosis unless the data base indicates otherwise. For example, if it is documented that the patient is already knowledgeable about the signs and symptoms, influencing factors, and complications of the problem, then this expected outcome need not be included in the care plan.

2. All expected outcome statements must have a time frame stated in terms of visits or weeks. The time frame is a "guestimate" and may be changed with documented rationale when found to be unrealistic.

3. Outcome criteria that do not apply to an individual patient should be deleted from the care plan. However, there must be at least two criteria under each outcome statement.

4. Where slashes are used in the printed outcome statements and criteria, the nurse is to choose whichever word(s) are most appropriate for the plan of care.

5. The expected outcome level chosen for each nursing diagnosis is based upon severity of each problem identified. For example, the patient may exhibit Level I impaired mobility (fracture) concurrent with Level III decreased cardiac output.

6. Once an outcome level is chosen for a nursing diagnosis, the outcome statements and criteria must be selected from that level. For example, a patient with Level II impaired skin integrity requires Level II outcome statements and criteria.

7. In developing the nursing care plan, the care plan should be modified to reflect the uniqueness of each patient's situation.

FIGURE 3
Example of Outcome Statement and Criteria

IMPAIRMENT OF SKIN/MUCOSA/TISSUE INTEGRITY RELATED TO: _____

Outcome Statement/Criteria

Level I	Level II	Level III
Patient demonstrates knowledge related to impaired skin/mucosa/tissue integrity.	*Patient/caregiver demonstrates knowledge related to impaired skin/mucosa/tissue integrity.*	*Patient/caregiver demonstrates knowledge related to severe impairment in skin/mucosa/tissue integrity.*
• Identifies sign/symptoms of impaired skin/mucosa/tissue integrity • Identifies factors that influence impaired skin/mucosa/tissue integrity • Identifies potential sequelae/complications of impaired skin/mucosa/tissue integrity	• Identifies sign/symptoms of impaired skin/mucosa/tissue integrity • Identifies factors that influence impaired skin/mucosa/tissue integrity • Identifies potential sequelae/complications of impaired skin/mucosa/tissue integrity	• Identifies signs/symptoms of impaired skin/mucosa/tissue integrity • Identifies factors that influence impaired skin/mucosa/tissue integrity • Identifies potential sequelae/complications of impaired skin/mucosa/tissue integrity
Patient identifies/demonstrates measures to prevent/correct impaired skin/mucosa/tissue integrity.	*Patient/caregiver identifies/demonstrates measures to control/correct impaired skin/mucosa/tissue integrity.*	*Patient/caregiver identifies/demonstrates measures to manage severe impairment in skin/mucosa/tissue integrity.*
• Demonstrates proper knowledge/administration of medications • Performs necessary treatments/procedures • Identifies sign/symptoms necessary to report to health care team • Identifies appropriate long-term follow-up plan of care • Identifies/utilizes appropriate community resources	• Demonstrates proper knowledge/administration of medications • Performs necessary treatments/procedures • Identifies signs/symptoms necessary to report to health care team • Identifies appropriate long-term follow-up plan of care • Identifies/utilizes appropriate community resources	• Demonstrates proper knowledge/administration of medications • Performs necessary treatments/procedures • Identifies signs/symptoms necessary to report to health care team • Identifies appropriate long term follow-up plan of care • Identifies/utilizes appropriate community resources
Patient achieves/maintains skin/mucosa/tissue integrity.	*Patient exhibits healing/control of impaired skin/mucosa/tissue integrity.*	*Patient exhibits healing/control of severe impairment in skin/mucosa/tissue integrity.*
• Absence of infection • Skin/mucosa/tissue intact	• Size reduction of lesion • Drainage reduction • Absence of infection • Development of granulation tissue	• Size reduction/absence of extension of lesion • Decreased drainage • Evidence of improving circulation to area • Absence/decreased infection

FIGURE 4
Example of Outcome Statements and Nursing Action Cues

IMPAIRMENT OF SKIN/MUCOSA/TISSUE INTEGRITY RELATED TO: _____

Expected Outcome Statements/Nursing Action Cues

Level I	Level II	Level III
A. *Patient demonstrates knowledge related to impaired skin/mucosa/tissue integrity within* _____ *visits.*	A. *Patient/caregiver demonstrates knowledge related to impaired skin/mucosa/tissue integrity within* _____ *visits.*	A. *Patient/caregiver demonstrates knowledge related to severe impairment in skin/mucosa/tissue integrity within* _____ *visits.*
10. Signs/symptoms	10. Signs/symptoms	10. Signs/symptoms
11. Influencing factors	11. Influencing factors	11. Influencing factors
12. Sequelae/complications	12. Sequelae/complications	12. Sequelae/complications
B. *Patient identifies/demonstrates measures to prevent/correct impaired skin/mucosa/tissue integrity within* _____ *visits.*	B. *Patient/caregiver identifies/demonstrates measures to control/correct impaired skin/mucosa/tissue integrity within* _____ *visits.*	B. *Patient/caregiver identifies/demonstrates measures to manage severe impairment in skin/mucosa/tissue integrity within* _____ *visits.*
10. Medications and side effects	10. Medications and side effects	10. Medications and side effects
11. Treatments and procedures	11. Treatments and procedures	11. Treatments and procedures
12. Signs/symptoms to report, including ER actions	12. Signs/symptoms to report, including ER actions	12. Signs/symptoms to report, including ER actions
13. Long-term follow-up plan of care	13. Long-term follow-up plan of care	13. Long-term follow-up plan of care
14. Community resources	14. Community resources	14. Community resources
15. Safety-related behaviors	15. Safety-related behaviors	15. Safety-related behaviors
C. *Patient achieves/maintains skin/mucosa/tissue integrity within* _____ *weeks.*	C. *Patient exhibits healing/control of impaired skin/mucosa/tissue integrity within* _____ *weeks.*	C. *Patient exhibits healing/control of severe impairment in skin/mucosa/tissue integrity within* _____ *weeks.*
10. Status of infection	10. Size of lesion	10. Size of lesion
11. Skin/mucosa/tissue status	11. Drainage	11. Drainage
	12. Status of infection	12. Status of infection
	13. Granulation tissue	13. Circulation to area

FIGURE 5
Example of Nursing Care Plan Format

VISITING NURSE ASSOCIATION OF METROPOLITAN DETROIT
NURSING CARE PLAN

NAME _____ CASE NUMBER _____ DO _____

DATE OF INITIAL PLAN _____ LEVEL I NURSE SIGNATURE _____

DATE E.O./ACTION ACHIEVED	NURSING DIAGNOSIS, EXPECTED OUTCOMES, PLAN & ACTIONS
	081 Impairment of Skin/Mucosa/Tissue Integrity Related to
	A. Patient demonstrates knowledge related to impaired skin/mucosa tissue integrity within visits.
	10. Signs/symptoms
	11. Influencing factors
	12. Sequelae/complications
	13. Pathophysiology of Disease Process
	B. Patient identifies/demonstrates measures to prevent/correct impaired skin/mucosa/tissue integrity
	within visits.
	10. Medications and side effects
	11. Treatments and procedures
	12. Signs/symptoms to report including ER actions
	13. Long term follow-up plan of care
	14. Community resources
	15. Safety related behaviors
	C. Patient achieves/maintains skin/mucosa/tissue integrity within weeks.
	10. Status of infection
	11. Skin/mucosa/tissue status
	12. Vital signs

K-113

Part 6

Functional Approaches

Evaluation
of a VNA Mental
Health Project

Pauline Vincent and Janet R. Price

This article represents an early effort to identify and quantify the out-comes of community-based mental health nursing services. It is also an example of a joint nursing research effort between academic and practice-based professionals.

This study evaluated the Mental Health Project (MHP) of the Visiting Nurse Association of Cleveland (VNA). The VNA has a generalized public health nursing program and has served the Greater Cleveland Area since 1902.

BACKGROUND OF THE STUDY

The MHP was initiated in July 1969 when the VNA obtained funds through the Cuyahoga County Community Mental Health and Retardation Board (CMHRB) to provide public health nursing services in the home for selected patients who had been discharged from four psychiatric hospitals. Cooperative

Reprinted with permission from *Nursing Research,* 26 (September-October 1977), copyright © 1977 *Nursing Research,* pp. 361–367.

agreements were established jointly by the participating hospitals and the VNA. The nursing service focused on helping referred patients adjust to their home and community environments, supervising treatment and medication regimens, and assisting patients' families with meeting their responsibilities for patient care.

During the first two years of this service, 616 psychiatric patients received VNA services, including coordination of patient care plans with the referring hospitals and other community agencies as well as home visits to implement these plans. At present, because funds for MHP are limited, the VNA makes only a specified number of visits to MHP patients each year.

This service to psychiatric patients needed to be examined to determine its effectiveness in relation to the stated MHP goals and to obtain more specific information about patients and services included in MHP. This information could be used as a base for subsequent decisions related to MHP, as well as for interpretation of the findings regarding the effectiveness of the service.

The opportunity to evaluate MHP arose when the University of North Carolina School of Public Health invited the VNA and the public health nursing faculty of Case Western Reserve University (CWRU) to participate in the Epidemiological Foundations of Evaluation Training Program from July 1971 through June 1973. With the approval of the CMHRB, a quasi-experimental design was chosen for the study.

Hypothesis

In conjuction with VNA district directors, the following hypothesis was selected to be tested: Visiting nurse services help to maintain or improve the social functioning and medical behaviors of patients discharged from psychiatric hospitals.

METHOD

Design

The study was designed so that the ratio of treatment group to control group patients would be two to one. In this way, fewer patients referred to the VNA would be assigned to the control group and, thus, not get VNA services. Beginning in March 1972, the names of all patients discharged from inpatient services and referred to the VNA by the participating psychiatric hospitals were channeled through the VNA main office. So that the patients would be assigned systematically on a random basis to the two study groups, the first two referred patients were assigned to the treatment group and the third was assigned to the control group, the next two were assigned to the treatment group and the sixth to the control group, and so on.

Treatment group patients received home visits from the staff nurses in whose area they resided. Those in the control group did not receive VNA services, unless extenuating circumstances affected this assignment during the study period. As agreed with the psychiatric hospitals, for this the extenuating circumstances included: need for home visits for the administration of medicines by injection, specific request for home visits by the VNA from the referring hospital after being informed within 48 hours of the patient's assignment to the control group, and specific request of a patient or family. A control group patient who received VNA services was automatically excluded from that group and the study.

Attempts were made from March through December 1972 to contact each referred patient as soon as possible after referral to VNA and to request participation in the study. When the appointment for the first interview was made, the patient was asked to have a relative or close friend (a significant other) present at the time of the visit, if at all possible, so that all forms could be completed. The patient was then told that an interviewer would return in six months to determine the patient's level of functioning. The interval for the second interview was influenced, in part, by time limitations of the training program. In addition, the interval seemed to be realistic in view of the findings of other studies[1] and VNA statistics which indicated that half of the psychiatric patients had been discharged by the end of six months of VNA services.

Variables

The dependent variables examined included patients' posthospital employment, social behavior, and regularity of following prescribed medication regimen. Social behavior was determined from responses to the selected Katz Adjustment Scales.[2] The scales include one set of forms (R2 and S2) which determine the level of performance of socially expected activities. The S2 form is a self-rating form for the patient. The R2 form is designed for the "significant other," but is otherwise identical to the S2 form. For example, on the S2 form, the first item is "helping with household chores"; it is "helps with household chores" on the R2 form. One possible response on the S2 form is "am doing some"; it is "doing some" on the R2.

The patients' reports on employment and on compliance with medication regimens were used to determine these two behaviors. The decision to use patients' reports for these two factors was influenced in part by the lack of resources and the time restrictions of the training program.

Information was obtained regarding age, education, marital status, occupation, race, sex, and the number of persons in the household. If the patient was not the head of the household, education and occupation of the head of the household were obtained since they were to be used to determine socioeconomic status (SES) according to the two-factor index of social position developed by Hollingshead.[3] In addition, data were obtained on factors suggested as possible intervening variables by VNA staff nurses: length of current hospital admission, number of previous psychiatric hospital admissions, frequency of psychiatric clinic visits during the six months following discharge, previous services from the VNA, helping services currently working with the patient other than the VNA, and nonpsychiatric medications being taken regularly.

Procedure

The interviewing was done by nurses who had had experience in public health nursing. Some of the interviewers were enrolled in the CWRU graduate program in public health nursing; others were former VNA staff nurses. Group sessions were held to explain the purpose of the study to the interviewers, to review the method of structured interviews, and to discuss any anticipated problems.

To determine the effectiveness of VNA services, the two groups were compared according to reported employment, compliance with medication regimen, and level of performance of socially expected activities. Employment was examined from three aspects: employed during the year preceding this hospital admission, at the time of the first interview, during the six months following this discharge.

Each respondent was asked what psychiatric medications he was taking, if they had been prescribed, how often the doctor said they should be taken, and how often the respondent "*missed* taking your nerve pills (psychiatric medicines) during the past two weeks." Only oral medications were included; pro re nata medications were excluded. Based on respondents' reports, each medication was scored on a five-point Likert-type scale that ranged from "always" to "never." The definitions for these categories were similar to those used by Michaux et al.[4] For purposes of this analysis, the "rarely" through "always" responses were categorized as "missed." Only those who reported that they never missed taking *any* of the prescribed medications were recorded in the "never" category. Therefore, if a respondent reported that he "never missed" taking one medication, but did miss taking a second medication "some of the time," that was recorded as "missed."

To determine level of performance of socially expected activities at the time of discharge and six months later, each respondent was asked to indicate whether he was "not doing," "doing some," or "doing regulary" each of the 16 activities listed. A score of one was given for each item the respondent indicated he was "not doing." "Doing some" was scored two, and "doing regularly" was scored three. Therefore, the possible range of scores was from 16 to 48. The items ranged from "dress and take care of myself" and "remember to do important things" to "get along with family members," "entertain friends at home," and "support the family."

Findings were subjected to chi-square analysis, and significance level was set at .05.

FINDINGS

During the period of the study, 254 patients were referred to the VNA. More than half (58 percent) were female, and the control group had a larger proportion of females. Race of more than half (54 percent) was nonwhite, but the proportion of nonwhite in the control group was greater than in the treatment group (Table 1). Age range was from 15 to 87 years among the 251 for whom this information was available. The average age for the treatment group was 42.3 years, and 40.0 years for the control group.

TABLE 1
Patients Referred and Study Respondents According to Sex, Race, and Study Group (in Number and Percent)

	Patients Referred						Respondents					
	Study Group						Study Group					
	Treatment		Control		Total		Treatment		Control		Total	
Variable	N	%	N	%	N	%	N	%	N	%	N	%
Sex												
Male	75	45	31	36	106	42	31	41	17	49	48	44
Female	94	55	54	64	148	58	44	59	18	52	62	56
Total	169	100	85	100	254	100	75	100	35	100	110	100
Race												
White	87	51	29	34	116	46	38	51	9	26	47	43
Nonwhite	82	49	55	66	137	54	37	49	26	74	63	57
Total	169	100	84[a]	100	253	100	75	100	35	100	110	100

[a] Race for one control patient was not known.

When contacted for the first interview, 162 patients agreed to participate. The 92 who were lost to the study included 61 from the treatment group and 31 from the control group (Table 2). The most frequent reasons for losses from the first and second interviews were: interviewers were unable to locate patients, patients refused to participate, patients were not taken under care by the visiting nurses, patients had been readmitted to a psychiatric hospital, and control patients required home visits. Other reasons included exclusion because the patients were outpatient department referrals, were living in sponsor homes, were in a medical hospital, had died, or were in jail.

TABLE 2
Referred Patients Lost to the Study by Study Group and by Sex and Race (in Number and Percent)

	Study Group					
	Treatment		Control		Total	
Variable	N	%	N	%	N	%
Sex						
Male	30	49	9	29	39	42
Female	31	51	22	71	53	58
Total	61	100	31	100	92	100
Race						
White	34	56	16	55	50	55
Nonwhite	27	44	14	45	41	45
Total	61	100	30[a]	100	91	100

[a] Race for one control patient was unknown.

This first report of the findings focuses on only the 110 patients who reported on their level of performance of socially expected activities (Form S2) and completed both interviews (Table 3). As 254 patients were referred to VNA during the study, the 110 patients included in this report constituted 43 percent of the total referred.

TABLE 3
Patients by Study Group for Whom Complete Information Was Available (in Number and Percent)

	Study Group		
Category	Treatment	Control	Total
S2 forms and both inter-views	75	35	110
S2 and R2 forms and both interviews[b]	39[a]	26[a]	65[a]
Forms incomplete[c]	20	32	52
Total	95	67	162

[a] This subcategory does not contribute to the total.

[b] R2 (significant other report) and S2 (self-report) forms measured socially expected activities.

[c] This category includes those who did not complete forms on first and/or second interviews.

Of the 110 patients who gave information on S2 forms and both inter-views, approximately two-thirds ($N = 75$) were in the treatment group. There was no significant difference between treatment and control groups accord-ing to sex, marital status, SES, or household size. In both groups more than one-third reported they had never married, about one-fifth were married at the time of the interview, more than 90 percent of the households were categorized as being in the two lowest SES levels. More than half the patients in each group were living with two or more persons; the range of household sizes extended to 15. Eleven treatment group patients reported living in households with six or more persons, compared with four control group patients reporting this; no control group patient reported living with more than nine other persons (Table 4).

TABLE 4
Respondents (N = 110) According to Household Size (in Number and Percent)

	Study Group			
	Treatment		Control	
Number in Household	N	%	N	%
One	14	18.7	2	5.7
Two	20	26.6	7	20.0
Three to six	30	40.0	22	62.8
More than six	11	14.7	4	11.5
Total	75	100.0	35	100.0

Treatment and control groups differed significantly ($p = .05$) according to age and race. The age range for the treatment group extended from 17 to 82 years, with an average of 41.9 years; for the control group, the range was 15 to 54 years, with an average of 33.8 years ($t = 2.65$, $df = 108$). Slightly more than half the treatment group were white, compared with slightly more than one-fourth in the control group ($chi\text{-}square = 6.07$, $df = 1$) (see Table 1).

Regarding employment, a smaller proportion of treatment group members was employed in each category (Table 5). Only 9 percent of the treatment group reported that they were employed at the time of the first interview, compared with 31 percent of the control group. This difference between the two groups was significant ($chi\text{-}square = 8.50$, $df = 1$, $p = .01$), but decreased in the six months. The proportion of control group members employed remained the same from the first to the second interview, whereas the employment rate increased 14 percent in the treatment group.

TABLE 5
Employment Data of Respondents (N = 110) by Study Group (in Number and Percent)

	Employed					
	Before Hospital Admission		After Hospital Discharge		During 6-Month Period	
Study Group	N	%	N	%	N	%
Treatment	27	36	7	9	17	23
Control	16	46	11	31	11	31

In comparing the groups according to reported frequency at which they missed taking medications, 26 of the 110 respondents were deleted because no oral psychiatric medications were prescribed for 7 treatment and 3 control respondents, according to their reports, and information was not available on the 12 treatment and 4 control patients who were in psychiatric hospitals at the time of the second interview. The proportion of patients in the treatment group who reported that they "never" missed taking their psychiatric medications was higher than the proportion in this group who reported they did miss taking them, and was higher than the proportion in the control group who reported they "never" missed taking them, but did not reach significance (Table 6).

TABLE 6
Respondents (N = 110) by Group Who Reported Psychiatric Medications Missed (in Number and Percent)

Missed Medications	Group					
	Treatment[a]		Control[b]		Total	
	N	%	N	%	N	%
Never	36	64	12	43	48	57
Yes	20	36	16	57	36	43
Total	56	100	28	100	84	100

[a] Excludes 12 hospitalized patients and 7 who had none prescribed.

[b] Excludes 4 hospitalized patients and 3 who had none prescribed.

Little difference was noted between the two groups regarding kind and number of psychiatric medicines they reported had been prescribed. However, a higher proportion in the treatment group (69 percent) than in the control group (51 percent) had medication supervision as a stated reason for referral. An additional difference between the groups in relation to medication was that no control group patients were on intramuscular Prolixin® whereas 12 in the treatment group received it. Six patients were excluded from the control group and the study since this injection required visiting nurse services. The intramuscular administration of Prolixin® , is most often prescribed for noninstitutionalized psychiatric patients who either are unable to take oral medications or are known to have been irregular in their taking of oral medications.

Little difference was noted between treatment and control groups in their level of performance of socially expected activities. Scores for the treatment group at the time of the first interview ranged from 19 to 41, with a mean of 31.68. For the control group the range was 19 to 46, with a mean of 31.57. Without the scores of the patients hospitalized at the time of the second interview, the average of the second scores was 31.71 for the treatment group, 31.40 for the control group when they were adjusted for age and race.

When the selected intervening variables were examined, in general minimal differences were identified between the treatment and control groups: 20 percent of the treatment group and 11 percent of the control group reported on the first interview that their most recent psychiatric hospital admission had been more than three months in length. The median category for the length of this hospital admission was one to three months for both groups. This category included 36 percent of the treatment group and 46 percent of the control group. The range was from less than one week to 11 years.

According to their reports, 43 percent of each group had had more than three psychiatric hospital admissions. The median number for each group was three, with a range that extended to 13 admissions to psychiatric hospitals prior to their first interview for this study.

Forty-four of the 75 treatment group (59 percent) and 18 of the 35 control group (55 percent) reported that they had made monthly psychiatric clinic visits during the first three months following the first interview. These percentages decreased to 49 percent for each group during the second three months, during which time 13 percent of the treatment group and 19 percent of the control group reported that they had made no psychiatric clinic visits. Two treatment group patients reported making weekly clinic visits during the first three months, but none reported this for the second three months. No control group patients reported they had made weekly clinic visits the first three months, but one did indicate making weekly clinic visits during the second three months.

Seventeen (23 percent) of the treatment group and 8 (23 percent) of the control group had received VNA services previous to their most recent hospital admission. There were 29 (39 percent) in the treatment group and 10 (29 percent) in the control group who reported receiving supportive services that would supplement or supplant VNA services during the six months following the first interview; 23 (31 percent) of the treatment group and 8 (23 percent) of the control group reported receiving supportive services from social caseworkers. Other services received included homemaker services at home and day care center services. Both patients who reported receiving homemaker services were in the treatment group.

Information was obtained regarding prescribed nonpsychiatric medications taken regularly on the premise that this would be an indicator of physical medical problems that might be of concern to the patients and would present additional activities at the patients would have to remember to do. Nineteen (25 percent) of the treatment group and 4 (11 percent) of the control group reported they were regularly taking prescribed nonpsychiatric medications. The conditions for which they were taking the medications included infections, diabetes, epilepsy, parkinsonism, and thyroid disorders. The information was not available on the 12 treatment and 4 control group patients who were in psychiatric hospitals at the time of the second interview.

Calculating the difference between the remaining 63 treatment group and 31 control group respondents, according to their taking of these medications, the difference between the two groups was not significant.

DISCUSSION

As several authors indicated and demonstrated, program evaluation studies and laboratory experimental studies differ markedly in the number of factors over which the investigators have control.[6] This is particularly apparent when the evaluation study includes interviews of noninstutionalized subjects. In this study of discharged psychiatric patients, 92 of the 254 patients were lost to the study initially. This 36.2 percent loss is equal to the proportion of discharged psychiatric patients who did not complete test I in the study reported by Michaux et al.[7] Of the 139 in their study who completed test I, 91 patients (65.5 percent) completed a sufficient number of tests to be included in their final report. This percentage was slightly less than the 67.8 percent who were included in this report of the VNA referrals (i.e., 110 of the 162 who completed the first interview).

Of particular concern in regard to the losses is the fact that the largest number were in the category of "unable to locate." Of the 254 patients referred to the VNA the interviewers were unable to contact 24 at the addresses given by the referring hospital or elsewhere, in spite of extensive efforts. This nine percent loss is somewhat comparable to the 11 percent that Spiegel and Younger reported in their study of discharged psychiatric patients; of the 725 questionnaires they sent, 84 did not reach their destination because the patient was no longer at the address supplied by the hospital from which they were discharged and no forwarding addresses were available.[8] This finding raises questions regarding the accuracy of hospitals' address records and how hospitals maintain contact with the patients they discharge. It also suggests additional, and perhaps unnecessary, problems and costs to agencies such as the VNA to which these patients are referred for postdischarge services.

In view of the methodologic problems inherent in this kind of evaluation study, only tentative general conclusions can be drawn. For example, a higher percentage in the treatment group obtained employment during the six-month period following discharge than in the control group. Although the difference was not statistically significant, treatment group patients were more likely to be taking their prescribed psychiatric medications than were control group patients. Only on socially expected activities were the two groups almost equal.

Data on Taking Prescribed Medications

In interpreting the data on the taking of medications, several factors should be considered. The treatment group may have had a negative bias (or disadvantage) in this comparison because, in part, of the design of the study. All six control group patients for whom intramuscular Prolixin® was prescribed were automatically excluded. The 12 treatment group patients for whom this medication was prescribed remained in the study. Since this is most often prescribed for problem patients, the treatment group may have been biased on this factor. Support for this is suggested by the finding that a higher proportion of the treatment group than the control group had been referred for medication supervision.

The proportion of control group patients who reported they were not taking their medications as prescribed was 57 percent. This finding was similar to several studies based on patients' reports which had a predominance of respondents over 30 years of age and who had long-term chronic conditions. Studies which included respondents in these categories and which had similar findings have been reported by Neely and Patrick, Schwartz, et al., and Vincent.[9] By comparison, the report of 36 percent of treatment group subjects, who had had medications prescribed and were not taking them as prescribed, was less then the percentages in these cited studies. In none of these cited studies were visiting nurses making regular home visits to encourage the patients to follow their medical regimens.

Scores for Socially Expected Activities

The two groups had almost equal averages on their scores for socially expected activities at the time of the first and at the time of second interviews. In view of the significant difference between the two groups according to the socially expected activity of employment, the lack of difference between the scores of the groups seems to be a discrepancy. Several factors may help explain this apparent discrepancy.

The limitation of only three answer choices on the instrument might have influenced results.[10] A respondent with a score of two for an item on the first and second interviews might actually have demonstrated a progression in that particular activity. For example, a patient might indicate he was doing "some" in response to "dress and take care of myself" on the first interview, and yet be doing this as infrequently as once a week. Unless he were doing this "regularly" at the time of the second interview, his score would continue to be two on this item.

According to some VNA staff nurses, it may take a few months of regular visiting to achieve the goal of having the patients verbally express themselves. One staff nurse visited a catatonic schizophrenic patient for more than two months before verbal interchanges occurred to any degree. This patient usually remembered when the nurse was to visit, and might have a score of two on the item "remember to do important things" on the first interview. Although progress in this activity might be demonstrated in six months, this patient's score would remain at two unless she reported that she was "doing regularly" this activity.

A second factor was that the patients who were referred to the VNA might have been too homogenous in their level of social adjustment for this particular instrument to discriminate differences that might have occurred. The Katz Adjustment Scales were found to "discriminate between groups who were quite different in over-all adjustment."[11] However, the possible homogeneity of treatment and control groups is suggested by the following: more than 90 percent of each group were in the lower socioeconomic classes, more than 60 percent of each group were schizophrenic, more than 55 percent of each group had three or more psychiatric hospital admissions, and more than 60 percent of each group were referred by one state psychiatric hospital.

A third factor is related to the average scores of slightly more than 31 on performance for both the treatment and control groups. These scores fell in the "unfavorable" category of the one-year study of postdischarged psychiatric patients reported by Michaux et al. At no time during their one-year study did the "non-relapsers" have a score below 35.4; the average score of the "non-relapsers" at six months following discharge was 36.4. Among the "relapsers" who had been readmitted to psychiatric hospitals during the year of the study, the average score at the end of the year was 33.8. The investigators stated scores of 34 or less would be "unfavorable."

Additional Predictor Characterisitics

In this study patients had additional characteristics which Michaux and his associates considered "unfavorable" or predictors of poor adjustment. These predictors include: never married, diagnosis of schizophrenia, three or more prior admissions to a psychiatric hospital, and less than a tenth grade education. The treatment and control groups had sizable proportions of each of these characteristics. In the treatment group, 29 (39 percent) never married, 32 (43 percent) had less than a tenth grade education, 46 (61 percent) had three or more prior admissions, and 48 (64 percent) were schizophrenic. In the control group, 14 (40 percent) never married, 13 (37 percent) had less than a tenth grade education, 20 (57 percent) had three or more prior admissions, and 26 (74 percent) were shcizophrenic. Additional characteristics that might be presumed to be "unfavorable" are diagnoses of alcoholism and drug addiction, mental deficiency, organic brain disorders, as well as physical handicaps that might "preclude reasonably adequate social functioning,"[12] This presumption is based on the fact that psychiatric patients with these characteristics were excluded from their study. They were not excluded from this study. Twelve in the treatment group and five in the control group had been referred with diagnoses of addiction or organic brain disorder.

Data on Readmissions

Although the proportion of treatment group subjects in psychiatric hospitals at the time of the second interview was larger than that of control group subjects, it should not be concluded that patients who received VNA services were more likely to be readmitted. In fact, the data suggested the opposite position. Fewer treatment group (28 percent) than control group (34 percent) respondents reported they were readmitted to psychiatric hospitals within six months of their first interview.

The proportions of readmissions within the treatment group and within the control group were somewhat higher than those of other reported studies. For example, 22 percent of the 139 discharged psychiatric patients who completed test I in the Michaux et al. study had at least one readmission within six months of their discharge.[13] Similar proportions were reported by Pasamanick et al. and by Spiegel and Younger.[14] Why the proportions of readmissions among the treatment and control groups in the present study were higher than these cited studies is difficult to determine.

Another possible reason for the differences between the proportion of readmissions within the treatment group and the other studies was suggested by the frequency of home visits to the schizophrenic patients in the Pasamanick et al. study. The public health nurses who were part of their study staff visited the patients weekly during the first three months and then twice a month during the second three months folowing each patient's discharge. The nurses also delivered the prescribed psychiatric medications to the patients on each home visit. One can infer from the frequency of these home visits that the average number of visits made to the patients was slightly more than three per month. The average number of VNA visits made to the patients in this study was 2.3 per month. This finding raises the question of whether more frequent visits to the psychiatric patients might have decreased the percentage of readmissions. Without additional data, it is difficult to determine if the readmissions were prompted by early recognition by the VNA nurses of psychiatric difficulties or if the assistance needed by the patients in the community was not sufficient to meet their needs.

Adequacy of Community Resources

The question of the adequacy of community resources to meet the needs of discharged psychiatric patients was suggested also by the finding that only 39 percent of the treatment group and 29 percent of the control group reported receiving assistance from agencies other than the VNA. As Davis et al. concluded from their study, "schizophrenics, in order to remain successfully in the community, must have continuous supervision and medication...It remains for psychiatric or social care to prevent the social deterioration of patients."[15] Becker, Pasamanick et al., and Spiegel and Younger also argued for intensive and coordinated community services for psychiatric patients.[16]

To say the respondents in this study were not receiving additional services because they were not available, not acceptable, or not known is impossible with the data at hand. However, an average of 2.3 home visits a month and monthly visits to the psychiatric clinic do not seem to qualify as intensive services to patients who have "unfavorable" characteristics and the relatively low average of socially expected activities scores that this group of respondents had. Some VNA staff nurses had great difficulty in contacting the appropriate personnel at the psychiatric hospitals to obtain information or to foster continuity of care. Some had problems in obtaining supplementary assistance for their patients because many of their psychiatric patients are unable to get to other agencies for the services they have to offer—because of the capabilities of the patients and the difficulties and costs of transportation to get to the resources. With few exceptions, only the VNA has services that are provided in the patients' homes.

The value of public health nursing services to psychiatric patients in the community is not questioned, and the hypothesis formulated for this evaluation was supported. The report of the Cooperative Care Project by the New Haven Visiting Nurse Association concluded that "public health nursing has a significant role to play" in the aftercare of psychiatric patients.[17] Pasamanick et al. selected public health nurses as principal participants in their controlled study to determine the efficacy of home care for schizophrenic patients in part because "the public health nurse, by virtue of her training and experience and traditional service activities as friend, counselor, advisor, general supporter, observer, and informant on patient and family life, is uniquely equipped to function in a home care mental health program."[18] Others have expressed similar positions. However, none has suggested that public health nurses should be the only assistance available to these patients.

The complexity of and frequently long-standing problems of psychiatric patients suggest the need for coordinated services of public health nurses and a variety of disciplines and agencies.[19]

ABOUT THE AUTHORS

At the time of writing, Pauline Vincent, RN, was Associate Director in Administration, Visiting Nurse Association of Cleveland, Ohio. At the time this study was done, she was Associate Professor of public health nursing, Western Reserve University, Cleveland. Janet R. Price was Executive Director, Visiting Nurse Association of Cleveland.

REFERENCES

1. W. W. Michaux, et al. *First Year Out* (Baltimore, MD: Johns Hopkins Press, 1969); and Benjamin Pasamanick, et al., *Schizophrenics in the Community* (New York: Appleton-Century-Crofts, 1967).

2. M. M. Katz and S. B. Lyerly, "Methods for Measuring Adjustment and Social Behavior in the Community: Part 1," *Psychological Reports,* 13(2) (1963), 503–535.

3. A. Hollingshead, *Two-Factor Index of Social Position,* New Haven, CT, 1957 (mimeographed).

4. Michaux et al., *First Year Out.*

5. A. Di Mascia and R. I. Shader, eds., *Clinical Handbook of Psychopharmacology* (New York: Jason Aronson, 1970).

6. P. H. Rossi and Walter Williams, eds., *Evaluating Social Programs* (New York: Academic Press, 1972; H. C. Schulberg, et al., *Program Evaluation in the Health Field* (New York: Behavioral Publications, 1969); E Suchman, *Evaluative Research* (New York: Russell Sage Foundation, 1968); and C. H. Weiss, *Evaluation Research* (Englewood Cliffs, NJ: Prentice-Hall, 1972).

7. Michaux et al., *First Year Out.*

8. D. Spiegel and J. B. Younger, "Life Outside the Hospital," *Mental Hygiene,* 56 (Spring 1972), 9–20.

9. Elizabeth Neely and M. L. Patrick, "Problems of Aged Persons Taking Medications at Home," *Nursing Research,* 17 (January-February 1968), 52–55; Doris Schwartz, et al., *The Elderly Ambulatory Patient* (New York: Macmillan Co., 1964); and Pauline Vincent, "Factors Influencing Patient Noncompliance: A Theoretical Approach," *Nursing Research,* 20 (November-December 1971), 509–516.

10. Support for this statement was demonstrated in a study done to determine the reliability of the Mental Health Patient Assessment Record, which was developed by the VNA subsequent to the evaluation study. M. L. Stricklin, "The Inter-Observer Reliability of the Mental Health Patient Assessment Record," unpublished master's thesis, Case Western Reserve University, Cleveland, OH, 1976.

11. Michaux et al., *First Year Out,* 7.

12. Ibid., 8.

13. Ibid.

14. Pasamanick et al., *Schizophrenics in the Community;* and Spiegel and Younger, "Life Outside the Hospital."

15. A. E. Davis, et al., "Prevention of Hospitalization in Schizophrenia: Five Years after an Experimental Program," *American Journal of Orthopsychiatry,* 42 (April 1972), p. 387.

16. R. E. Becker, "Organization and Management of Community Mental Health Services," *Community Mental Health Journal,* 8 (November 1972), 292–302; Pasamanick et al., *Schizophrenics in the Community;* and Spiegel and Younger, "Life Outside the Hospital."

17. *The Role of Public Health Nursing in the After-Care of the Psychiatric Patient* (New Haven, CT: New Haven Visiting Nurse Association, 1966), 51.

18. Pasamanick et al., *Schizophrenics in the Community,* 59.

19. A. F. Beasley, et al., "The Follow-Up of Discharged Mental Patients by the Public

Health Nurse," *American Journal of Psychiatry,* 116 (March 1960), 834–837; Abraham Laurie and Gary Rosenberg, "Problems in Community Organization for Mental Health," *Hospital & Community Psychiatry,* 23 (November 1972), 350–353; and H. G. Lindberg and C. H. Branch, "Community Health Nursing in the Changing Mental Health Scene," *Journal of Nursing Administration,* 3 (November-December 1973), 41–44.

Using a Level of Function Scale (LORS-II) to Evaluate the Success of Inpatient Rehabilitation Programs

Emil J. Posavac and Raymond G. Carey

This article briefly describes a functional status tool used by rehabilitation professionals. Although developed for use in a rehabilitation facility, the LORS-II offers potential as a multidisciplinary evaluation tool for rehabilitation services provided in the home.

Concern about the evaluation of rehabilitation services is growing rapidly. This growth is seen in the development of program evaluation standards by the Commission on the Accreditation of Rehabilitation Facilities (CARF), the publication of articles on evaluation in rehabilitation and hospital journals, and the formation of a journal for evaluators in rehabilitation settings called the *Journal of the Organization of Rehabilitation Evaluators.*[1] This article describes several purposes of program evaluation and illustrates one approach to the evaluation of inpatient rehabilitation services.

The evaluation of services is a complex process; different kinds of rehabilitation facilities require different approaches to evaluation. For example, inpatient programs have needs that are different from outpatient programs. Furthermore, among inpatient programs, those serving a large proportion of patients who have

Reprinted with permission from *Rehabilitation Nursing*, 7 (November-December 1982), copyright © 1982, *Rehabilitation Nursing,* pp. 17-19.

had cerebrovascular accidents (CVAs) may focus on different behaviors than those programs serving primarily young accident victims. In addition, different types of evaluations can be done. For example, the need to implement an accountability system requires an approach that is different from the approach required when an overall view of the achievements of patients is desired.

When an accountability program is needed, the system described by Quigley can be considered.[2] Quigley reported on a system designed to: (1) increase the level of detail of patient records, (2) improve the accuracy of charts, (3) identify problems in the nursing patient care plan, (4) help in the nurses' advocacy role on behalf of patients by documenting need, (5) document patient progress. One advantage of this approach is that patient information is arranged in an easy-to-use format. However, the Quigley plan calls for 129 ratings of patient ability to be made each day. At three points during a patient's stay, 67 additional ratings are needed. There is concern by the authors as to whether staff members could really make so many ratings on each patient, day after day, without becoming perfunctory and casual. Nevertheless, the approach may well meet the goals that Quigley set out to achieve.

Another evaluation goal that an administrator or a clinician can consider is obtaining an overview of inpatients' success in regaining self-care or mobility independence. Gaining such an overview was the motivation behind the development of the Level of Rehabilitation Scale-II (LORS-II). This instrument, a revision of an earlier approach,[3] meets the CARF suggestions of a cost-effective approach to measuring the outcome of inpatient rehabilitation services because a small number of ratings are required to use the instrument, although many aspects of each patient's function are covered.

BRIEF DESCRIPTION OF LORS-II

LORS-II is described at some length in another medical journal.[4] The philosophy behind its specific format is presented in a new journal for rehabilitation evaluation.[5] Therefore, only a brief description of the instrument is presented here. LORS-II includes ratings of patient function on activities of daily living (ADL), mobility, and communication. Communication is divided into three components: (1) audible communication (speaking and listening), (2) written communication (reading and writing), (3) gestural communication. The ratings are made on five-point scales ranging from zero (patient does not perform the function) through four (patient performs the function reliably and independently). Figure 1 is the form used to record discharge level of function. Similar forms are used at admission and follow-up. The individual ratings are converted into percentages of perfect scores. Patients are only rated on those functional behaviors for which they receive therapy.

FIGURE 1
LORS-II Discharge Rating Form

Patient _____ Discharge Date: _____

    ID # _____

DISCHARGE RATINGS

Activities of Daily Living

                           Rating by:

	RN	OT	**Scoring:**
A. Dressing	☐	☐	Range = 0-4
B. Grooming	☐	☐	No therapy provided = 9
C. Washing/bathing	☐	☐	
D. Toileting	☐	☐	**Rater codes:**
E. Feeding	☐	☐	RN = Rehabilitation nurse
			OT = Occupational therapist
			PT = Physical therapist
			ST = Speech therapist

Mobility
(Check and rate one:)

	RN	PT
Ambulation (if possible) 1. ☐	☐	☐
Wheelchair management 2. ☐		

Communication

Verbal

	RN	ST
A. Auditory comprehension	☐	☐
B. Oral expression	☐	☐

	RN	ST
Gestural	☐	☐

Written

	ST
A. Reading comprehension	☐
B. Written expression	☐

Standard procedures call for nurses and approrpiate therapists to rate patients at admission and discharge. Spouses or adult children provide ratings at the 90-day follow-up. Former patients themselves provide the follow-up assessments when they are able to, as is the case for amputees.

NORMS FOR LORS-II

The authors stress that rehabilitation program evaluation is enhanced through using standard evaluation measures for which norms are available.

This report includes illustrative norm information that goes beyond information published previously and is presented in a different, perhaps more easily used format. Tables 1 and 2 contain norm information for the ADL scale for CVA patients. The mean age of the patients was 69 years. They were treated at private hospitals, one in a suburban setting and a smaller one in a semirural setting. Table 1 provides the expected levels of ADL function at discharge for 101 CVA patients with left hemisphere involvement. Table 2 provides the same information for 92 CVA patients with right hemisphere involvement. There are two parts to Table 2 because age is empirically related to the improvement of right CVA patients but is not related for left CVA patients. At this time, the reason why older CVA patients show less progress than young CVA patients when the right hemisphere is involved but not when the left hemisphere is involved is not fully understood.

These norms are not presented as final or definitive. More assessments are being gathered, and refinements in the norms will be made. However, providing norms for an instrument to assess progress in rehabilitation, although seldom done, can be helpful.

One way to use the tables is to enter the admission level column at the mean admission level of the patients treated and to note the expected ranges of discharge levels. The tables were constructed so that, on the average 25 percent of patients will be discharged in each of the four categories. The labels "Excellent," "Good," "Fair," and "Poor," are based on the 25th, 50th and 75th discharge percentiles at each level of admission. For right CVA patients, the tabled values must be corrected for patients' age. For example, according to Table 2, the "good" range for 70-year-old right CVA patients admitted at an ADL of 40 would be halfway between 70-81 (the "good"

TABLE 1
Levels of ADL at Discharge for 101 Left CVA Patients as Measured Using LORS-II

| Admission Level | Discharge Level | | | |
	Poor	Fair	Good	Excellent
85 - 94	*	*	*	*
75 - 84	*	*	*	*
65 - 74	65 - 80	81 - 92	93 - 100	*
55 - 64	55 - 72	73 - 84	85 - 96	97 - 100
45 - 54	45 - 64	65 - 77	78 - 88	89 - 100
35 - 44	35 - 57	58 - 69	70 - 81	82 - 100
25 - 34	25 - 49	50 - 61	62 - 73	74 - 100
15 - 24	15 - 42	43 - 54	55 - 66	67 - 100
5 - 14	5 - 34	35 - 46	47 - 58	59 - 100

*Very few patients are treated with admission levels this high.
Note: Twenty-five percent of left CVA patients are expected to be discharged in each of the four categories.

TABLE 2
Levels of ADL at Discharge Expected for 92 Right CVA Patients as Measured Using LORS-II

Admission Level	Discharge Level			
	Poor	Fair	Good	Excellent
Age 65				
85 - 94	*	*	*	*
75 - 84	*	*	*	*
65 - 74	65 - 83	84 - 95	96 - 100	*
55 - 64	55 - 74	75 - 86	87 - 98	99 - 100
45 - 54	45 - 66	67 - 78	79 - 90	91 - 100
35 - 44	35 - 57	58 - 69	70 - 81	82 - 100
25 - 34	25 - 48	49 - 60	61 - 72	73 - 100
15 - 24	15 - 39	40 - 51	52 - 63	64 - 100
5 - 14	5 - 30	31 - 42	43 - 54	55 - 100
Age 75				
85 - 94	*	*	*	*
75 - 84	*	*	*	*
65 - 74	65 - 79	80 - 91	92 - 100	*
55 - 64	55 - 70	71 - 82	83 - 94	95 - 100
45 - 54	45 - 61	62 - 73	74 - 85	86 - 100
35 - 44	35 - 52	53 - 64	65 - 76	77 - 100
25 - 34	25 - 44	45 - 56	57 - 68	87 - 100
15 - 24	15 - 35	36 - 47	48 - 59	60 - 100
5 - 14	5 - 27	28 - 38	39 - 50	51 - 100

*Very few patients are treated with admission levels this high.

Note: Twenty-five percent of right CVA patients are expected to be discharged in each of the four categories.

range for 65-year-old patients) and 65-76 (the "good" range for 75-year-old patients) or approximately 68-78.

A second way to use the tables is to enter the admission level column with an individual patient's admission level. Using the patient's discharge level, classify the patient's progress as "Poor," "Fair," "Good," or "Excellent." For example, using Table 1, progress of a left CVA patient admitted at 50 and discharged at 70 would be said to only be "Fair." Again, over time, 25 percent of patients are expected to be found in each category.

THE USE OF LORS-II IN PROGRAM MANAGEMENT

The information provided by LORS-II ratings and the norms can be used in several different ways. Some approaches are based on material gathered at different times in one facility, and other approaches use information from several facilities.

Lack of Meaningful Improvement

The first and most critical index to examine is patients' degree of improvement in the program. Clearly, patients who are provided rehabilitative therapy are expected to improve in their functional abilities. If improvment levels are so small that the improvement would go unnoticed by an observer, then the LORS-II values indicate that the staff needs to restructure the approach to care. Functional outcome values do not indicate where a problem may lie. A staff whose patients show minimal improvement would want to examine the breadth of services, the quality of services, and the communication among staff members.

Changes from Past Levels of Improvement

A program that documents successful outcomes with several patient samples but then discovers that patient improvement is markedly lower than baseline values should search for the reasons for decline. Lowered overall improvement may be due to several particularly dysfunctional patients in the program at the same time. However, continued lower levels of improvement seldom can be explained by unusual samples.

Another value of baseline data is apparent when significant improvements in care are instituted. The provision of new services is expected to result in improved outcomes. If new services lead to a change in the nature of patient population served, the norms are still valid because both admission and discharge levels are included in the norms. If more severely dysfunctional patients are treated, average admission levels will be lower; however, 25 percent of discharge levels is still expected in each of the four discharge categories listed in the tables.

Poor Relative Outcomes

A staff treating patients similar to those on which the tables were based would expect to find roughly similar levels of improvement among their patients. If patient improvement is markedly below that indicated by the tables, the staff would want to examine its services to learn whether improvements need to be made.

Goal Setting

One approach to evaluation in rehabilitation is to set goals for the degree of improvement by discharge. The illustrations in the CARF guide suggest that the staff indicate what percentages of patients are expected to achieve specified outcomes, namely the percentage of patients independent in dressing or feeding. However, realistic goals can be set for a program only after baseline assessments of improvement have been analyzed. Baseline information should be available before goals are set, because without such information, either overly ambitious or completely unchallenging goals may be chosen. Once baseline data are available, staff may initially set goals that match past experience and later raise them slightly. For example, instead of having 50 percent of patients falling in the good or excellent categories, a staff can raise the goal to 55 percent in these categories. Achieving goals through actual functional improvement and not through a more relaxed use of the rating instrument is important, whether it be the LORS-II or some other measure of functional ability. Maintaining a consistent interpretation of the scale is an important task for anyone supervising the evaluation of services.

SUMMARY

This article describes a method of using a functional behavior scale (LORS-II) in evaluating an inpatient facility treating CVA patients. Improvement norms for ADL are provided, and their use is illustrated. Evaluators of rehabilitation services can save considerable time by adopting an existing tool to assess patient progress and can conduct more sophisticated analyses using these norms. A quantitative assessment of the degree of patient progress permits the evaluation of improvements in quality of care.

ABOUT THE AUTHORS

At the time of writing, Emil J. Posavac, PhD, was Professor of Psychology, Loyola University of Chicago, Chicago, Illinois. Raymond G. Carey, PhD was Director, Health Care Evaluation Division, Parkside Medical Services Corporation, Park Ridge, Illinois.

REFERENCES

1. *Program Evaluation in Inpatient Medical Rehabilitation Facilities* (Tucson, AZ: Commission on the Accreditation of Rehabilitation Facilities, 1979); P. A. Quigley, "Nursing Evaluation in Rehabilitation," *ARN Journal*, 6(6) (1981), 12-14; and M. B. Swope, "Rehabilitation Can Use Joint Approach to Quality Assurance," *Hospitals*, October 1, 1981, 69-71.

2. Quigley, "Nursing Evaluation in Rehabilitation."

3. R. G. Carey and E. J. Posavac, "Program Evaluation of a Physical Medicine and Rehabilitation Unit: A New Approach," *Archives of Physical Medicine and Rehabilitation*, 59 (1978), 330-337.

4. R. G. Carey and E. J. Posavac, "Rehabilitation Program Evaluation Using a Revised Level of Rehabilitation Scale (LORS II)," *Archives of Physical Medicine and Rehabilitation* (1982).

5. E. J. Posavac and R. G. Carey, "Characteristics of Useful and Cost-Effective Methodologies of Outcome Evaluation in Rehabilitation Programs," *Journal of the Organization of Rehabilitation Evaluators*, 2(1) (1982), 19-27.

6. Ibid.; Carey and Posavac, "Program Evaluation of a Physical Medicine and Rehabilitation Unit"; and Carey and Posavac, "Rehabilitation Program Evaluation Using a Revised Level of Rehabilitation Scale."

Development and Use of Functional Client Outcome Measures

Mary Lou Christensen

In this previously unpublished piece, Christensen describes two outcome approaches used in Minnesota. The client outcome criteria represent locally developed standards based on the ANA Guidelines excerpted in Part I. The ADL Function Code tool offers an approach to functional outcome measurement. Both types of criteria are used, as Christensen describes, in a service agency.

Outcome measures of care provided to clients in the home are essential aspects of public health nursing practice. Specific outcome statements with their underlying behaviors not only indicate the progress the client has made by the end of the period during which services were provided, but also can serve as a guideline for the public health nurse for provision of service. Teaching about and observing those aspects of care and the client's status that are contained in the outcome criteria help the nurses' visits to be more purposeful and goal directed.

The client outcome criteria used in Ramsey County Public Health Nursing Service (RCPHNS) are based on original expected outcome criteria for clients that were developed in 1975 by peer groups of public health nurses from across Minnesota under the direction of the Minnesota Department of Health.[1] Since that time, RCPHNS staff have made major revisions of the criteria and identified new topic areas to meet their practice and documentation needs in the agency. As the revisions were completed and new topic areas of client outcome criteria developed, the completed products have been shared with the Minnesota Department of Health so that colleagues across the state can benefit from each others' work.[2]

An example of client outcome criteria—those for open wound situations that require dressing changes—is presented in Figure 1. The format for these care criteria include the basic elements of the client's knowledge or understanding of the situation, the management regime that has been developed, the extent to which psychosocial adjustments have been made, and the status of the client's condition or situation at discharge from service. This format is similar for all of the topics in the 12 sets of client outcome criteria being used in the agency.

In cases where the clients' physical functioning is of concern, the ADL Function Code (Fig. 2) is used. This assessment is done at both opening of the case and discharge from service. The public health nurse assesses the six functioning parameters of bathing, dressing, toileting, transferring, continence, and feeding on the independent (A column) or dependent (B or C columns) level, utilizing a separate sheet of descriptions that define the various levels of independence or dependence for each parameter. The pattern of the six checks falling across the grid, which represent the nurse's assessment, are then summarized by one of 14 mutually exclusive categories.

The example in Figure 2 represents a decline of functioning of seven categories in a terminally ill client prior to rehospitalization. Level 6C is identified at opening of the case and 2B at closure. Not only is the final outcome of physical functioning of the client documented at discharge from service, but the change in physical functioning from opening to closure is documented.

The ADL code is useful on a case-by-case basis for documenting a particular client's progress or decline in physical functioning. This information is placed in the computer and becomes part of the summary data kept for documentation of the client's health status. When totaled for a nurse's caseload, this summary data becomes useful for supervisors as a tool for analyzing the complexity of clients' physical functioning in her staff's caseload. For nursing administrators, the ADL code is helpful in describing in the aggregate the severity of clients' physical functioning and the amount of change that occurs in clients, from opening of the case to discharge from service by the staff. This information is used to describe agency caseloads in a summary manner to county commissioners and other funding sources.

ABOUT THE AUTHOR

Mary Lou Christensen, MPH, RN, is Associate Director, Ramsey County Public Health Nursing Service, St. Paul, Minnesota.

REFERENCES

1. See F. Decker, L. Stevens, M. Vancini, and L. Wedeking, "Using Patient Outcomes to Evaluate Community Health Nursing," *Nursing Outlook*, 27 (April 1979), 278-282. Reprinted in this volume, pp. xx-xx.

2. See *Outcome Criteria: Public Health Nursing Services and Home Health Care Services* (rev. ed.; Minneapolis: Minnesota Department of Health, Section of Public Health Nursing, October 1986). Excerpted in this volume, pp. xx-xx.

FIGURE 1
Example of Client Outcome Criteria

RAMSEY COUNTY PUBLIC HEALTH NURSING SERVICE

Client Outcome Criteria

Open Wound Requiring Dressing Change

Directions: Listed below are five core criteria and related behaviors descriptive of client outcomes for the population needing wound care. Please indicate by *date* in the appropriate column when *both behaviors* and *outcome criteria are met*. Use the *comments* column to describe *why outcomes have not been met*, or any other pertinent evaluative information, if desired. Use the bottom section to *state specific outcomes individualized* for this client's care plan.

Open Wound Criteria and Behaviors	Date Met Initials	Comments: If not met, why? etc.
1. Client and/or significant other understands healing process and its effects.		
a. Client and/or significant other describes cause of own wound.		
b. Client and/or significant other describes healing process of wound and/or complications of healing.		
c. Client and/or significant other relates healing process to own wound and prognosis of healing.		
2. Client and/or significant other understands management of healing process.		
a. Client and/or significant other states wound related medications or topical agents used and side effects of each.		
b. Client and/or significant other describes treatment and dressing changes utilizing principles of asepsis.		
c. Client and/or significant other describes the plan for use in possible complications of wound healing, i.e., odor, color change, increased pain, increased temperature, skin breakdown.		
d. Client and/or significant other verbalizes the significance of appropriate diet for wound healing.		
e. Client and/or significant other describes adjustments in activities to promote healing.		

FIG. 1 (continued)

Open Wound Criteria and Behaviors	Date Met Initials	Comments: If not met, why? etc.
3. Client and/or significant other implements a management program, independently as able.		
a. Client and/or significant other complies with medication regime.		
b. Client and/or significant other carries out treatment and dressing changes using principles of asepsis.		
c. Client has increased food intake from pre-wound status to achieve healing via protein, Vitamin C, and appropriate fluid content.		
d. Client adjusts activities to promote healing.		
4. Client accepts necessary life style adjustment.		
a. Client expresses positive/negative feelings about changed body image, drainage, pain or odor, and limitations it imposes.		
b. Client seeks and utilizes assistance through resources, if needed.		
c. Client maintains appropriate activity level.		
5. Client wound status.		
a. Redness, discharge, swelling or foul odor not present.		
b. Pain and tenderness in wound decreased.		
c. Depth and diameter of wound decreased.		
Specific Individualized Expected Outcomes Please List:		
1.		
2.		
3.		
4.		
5.		

FIGURE 2
Example of Completed ADL Function Code Form

RAMSEY COUNTY PUBLIC HEALTH NURSING SERVICE
ADL FUNCTION CODE

Step one: Based on your assessment using the descriptor sheet, place a check in whichever level box applies for each function.

	OPEN Level A	B	C		CLOSE Level A	B	C
Bathing			✓				✓
Dressing		✓				✓	
Toileting		✓				✓	
Transferring			✓				✓
Continence		✓					✓
Feeding	✓					✓	

Inde-pendence   Dependence   Inde-pendence   Dependence

Step Two: (Nurse responsibility)

Directions: Using grid in Step One as a guide, determine which one of the following categories applies and check the appropriate blank.

Open   Close

_____ _____ 8   Independent in feeding, continence, transferring, toileting, dressing, and bathing.

_____ _____ 7B   Dependent in one function which is at the B level.

_____ _____ 7C   Dependent in one function which is at the C level.

_____ _____ 6B   Dependent in bathing and one additional function of which at least one is at the B level.

_____ _____ 6C   Dependent in bathing and one additional function of which both are at the C level.

_____ _____ 5B   Dependent in bathing, dressing and one additional function of which 2 or more are at the B level.

_____ _____ 5C   Dependent in bathing, dressing and one additional function of which 2 or 3 are at the C level.

_____ _____ 4B   Dependent in bathing, dressing, toileting and one additional function of which 2 or more are at the B level.

_____ _____ 4C   Dependent in bathing, dressing, toileting and one additional function of which 3 or 4 are at the C level.

_____ _____ 3B   Dependent in bathing, dressing, toileting, transferring and one additional function of which 3 or more are at the B level.

_____ _____ 3C   Dependent in bathing, dressing, toileting, transferring and one additional function of which 4 or 5 are at the C level.

_____ _____ 2B   Dependent in all six functions of which 3 or more are at the B level.

_____ _____ 2C   Dependent in all six functions of which 4, 5 or 6 are at the C level.

_____ _____ 1   Dependent in at least two functions, but not classifiable in any other category.

Self-Management Outcome Criteria (SMOC) Record Form

Visiting Nurse and Home Care

The Self-Management Outcome Criteria (SMOC) tool presented here represents another local service agency's attempts to identify and quantify the impact of home health services on a client's functional status. Like the instruments described in Christensen, in the previous piece, the SMOC tool is used in conjunction with individual expected outcomes based on particular health problems. Both the Ramsey County Public Health Nursing Service ADL Function Code and the SMOC tool offer potential to measure outcomes in the aggregate. In each case, a summary score can be derived upon admission and a discharge rating can be predicted and then actually measured for evaluation purposes.

GUIDELINES FOR SMOC RECORD FORM

Purpose

- To promote an objective, quantitative, ongoing, systematic mechanism for documentation of a client's self-management level.
- To provide a clear, concise and consistent method for recording client self-management levels at time of admission and discharge.

- To assure the establishment of long-term goals (expected outcome levels) at time of admission.
- To provide a valid and reliable source of outcome data.

Rationale for Self-Management Framework

The primary objective of the agency, its personnel, and its services is "to enhance the capability of individuals, families, and communities to manage health and illness problems" (Visiting Nurse and Home Care, Inc., Bylaws and Objectives).

Definition of Self-Management

Self-management is defined as the *individual client's* ability to control his/her health and/or illness/disability problems within the home setting using his/her own resources and/or those of family/agency/community.

Five areas of self-management are identified (see Fig. 1):

I. *Level of Knowledge:* Any learning needed to improve or make self-management possible and safe.

II. *Reduction of Risks to Health:* Adaptation/personalization of daily routine and/or medical regimen to maximize improvement, stabilization, or maintenance of condition/situation as well as prevent deterioration/complications.

III. *Functional Ability/ADL Management:* Ability to perform all activities of daily living including those related to personal care, mobility within and outside of home, household maintenance, and business affairs.

IV. *Behavior-Mentation-Emotion (B-M-E):* Verbal and/or non-verbal behavior which delineates client's interactions with time, place, person, and self.

V. *Support from Significant Other(s) (SO):* Support includes physical and/or psychosocial assistance needed. Significant other includes a friend/family member/neighbor who would *usually* be expected to provide physical and psychosocial support as needed. *Medical/social services personnel* should not be considered as this significant person. *Remember:* Presence alone does not constitute support.

FIGURE 1
The Self-Management Outcome Criteria Tool

Visiting Nurse And Home Care, Inc.
SELF MANAGEMENT OUTCOME CRITERIA

Areas	CRITERION LEVELS			
	High			**Low**
	0	**1**	**2**	**3**
I. Level of Knowledge	Describes/demonstrates accurate application of knowledge/skills	States knowledge/ demonstrates skills with reinforcement/guidance/ supervision	Ready to learn but has -Limited/inaccurate knowledge -Difficulty with articulation/ application -Lack of confidence	Unable or unwilling to learn or apply knowledge. Lack of readiness (denies, disagrees with, or does not recognize need)
II. Reduction of risks to health	Minimizes risks associated with health/medical regimen. Adapts lifestyle/complies	Minimizes risks/complies with reinforcement/ guidance/supervision.	Risk avoidance/compliance vacillates or is questionable regardless of reinforcement/ guidance/supervision	Unable or unwilling to minimize risks/non-compliant Values conflict with medical regimen/preventive health principles
III. Functional ability/ADL management	Self-manages personal care, household duties, and business affairs	Self-manages but with diffi- culty	Manages with assistance only	Unable or unwilling to manage
IV. Behavior- Mentation- Emotion (B-M-E)	Social behavior appropriate Mental processes intact Manages stress Satisfying relationships/ activities/accomplishments Plans for future	Aware of and compensates for behavioral or mental pro- cess deviations most of the time Manages stress but with difficulty Ambivalent satisfaction with relationships/activities/ accomplishments Uncertain/ambivalent re: future plans	Awareness and/or compensation vacillates or is questionable Limited participation in and satisfaction with relationships/activities/ accomplishments Limited stress management and/or future planning	Unaware of deviations Unwilling or unable to compensate i.e. isolated, hostile, suicidal ideation, impaired mental processes, hopeless feelings, disoriented Relationships/activities are inappropriate, immature, unhealthy, dissatisfying, lacking, incomplete Future planning lacking, inappropriate, , unrealistic
V. Support from significant other(s) (s.o.)	Receives needed support from s.o.(s)	Receives needed support from s.o.(s) and community services/agencies	Receives needed support from community services/ agencies only	Unable or unwilling to use available supports Inappropriate use of supports Supports unavailable, insufficient, inconsis- tent, interfering, inappropriate, disruptive

EVALUATION DATA	DATE							
	AREAS	**Admission Level**	**Expected Level**					
	I Knowledge							
	II Risk Reduction							
	III FN/ADL							
	IV BME							
	V Support							
	Total							
	Evaluator							

*COMMENTS

Name:_____   Record Number:_____

VNA-C-100

Criterion Levels

Each area of self-management is sub-divided into four levels.

A descriptive statement is written for each level using outcome terminology (criterion level) (see Fig. 1).

Each criterion level is assigned a numerical level of 0, 1, 2, or 3.

Of the criterion levels, 0 represents the highest level of self-management and 3 represents the lowest. Criterion levels 1 and 2 represent gradations between the highest and lowest levels.

Each area of self-management is evaluated independently.

Operating Assumptions

As criterion level becomes closer to 0, client's ability to self-manage is increased.

As criterion level becomes closer to 3 (or 15 with total of 5 areas) client's ability to self-manage is decreased.

Direction of change of criterion level indicates direction of progress either positive (closer to 0), or negative (closer to 3 or 15).

Expected outcomes (goals) are mutually set with client.

Criterion levels are supported by other data in the record.

Self-management outcome criteria use does not substitute for need to use more specific outcome criteria (short-term goals) for areas such as physical status, learning, stress, etc., on flow sheet.

Relationship to Quality Assurance/Client Evaluation

For each area and overall self-management, practitioners and/or Quality Assurance Program Studies will be able to identify for each client and/or a target population of the following:

1. The admission level
2. The expected outcome level (long-term goal)
3. The degree and direction of level change expected
4. The discharge level
5. The actual degree and direction of level change between admission and discharge
6. The accuracy with which expected outcomes are predicted

7. The relationship(s) between the outcome levels and the process of care as documented

8. The relationship(s) between the outcome levels and profile factors.

Relationship to Record

1. The form is a permanent part of the record.

2. The ratings should be in agreement with other information in the record.

3. The form is placed on the right side of the record behind the Family Identification Sheet.

Accountability for Completion of Form

The *Client Care Coordinator* is ultimately accountable for the completion of this form. The responsibility may be delegated to another *professional* involved in the direct delivery of services to the client.

Must be completed for every client.

For a *child* who is too young to participate in self-management. The SMOC evaluation levels are done on the *primary caregiver*. Make sure that this information is clearly indicated. Put child's name at bottom of form. State under comment section that "Levels done on mother, father," etc.

Frequency of Evaluation

Admission Level.   *Must be completed as part of first visit. Serves as baseline.* Use "re-admit" when multiple admissions involved.

Expected Levels. *   *Must be completed as part of first visit* and with readmissions. Represents the *anticipated, final level* of the client's self-management (not illness) *at the time of discharge.* The expected level repesents the long term goals as mutually set by the client care coordinator and the client. May be re-done in conjunction with an Interim Level if condition/information changes significantly.

---

*Do *not* complete for one-visit admissions.

Interim Level.   *Must be completed once every 60 days.* Represents the evaluation of progress toward the Expected level. Documents a 60-day review of the client's current status which is required by State of Connecticut Home Care regulations.

Should be used to document levels when client is referred to hospital or physician and client service potentially may be terminated or a change in levels may be anticipated after a short interruption of service with record remaining open. If client is not returned to service this interim level can serve as the Discharge Level.

Discharge Level.   *Must be completed at time of last visit or telephone contact.* Provides the final evaluation of client's level of self-management as of the last visit or telephone contact. This level must reflect self-management—not illness level. Must be completed even when client dies, moves, refuses services, etc.

A System to Evaluate
Home Health Care Services

Elizabeth A. Daubert

Daubert's article describes an early attempt to measure the quality of home care services and focuses on the process of care. It is included here as a background document to the two articles that follow, written by Harris and others, which detail further development of this approach.

Home health agencies claim that their services meet a basic community need and that the quality of care they provide is of high caliber. Such statements paint a picture of a multi-service delivery system of unquestionable worth that functions in an appropriate, adequate, efficient, effective, and clinically competent manner. When evidence is sought to validate such statements, however, it soon becomes apparent that little hard data exist to substantiate such glowing claims.

In reality, most evaluations of community health nursing and other agency service components are based upon individual assumptions and preferences, not upon substantive evidence. One reason might be the absence of a satisfactory method of measuring the quality of care provided, not only by nursing but by each of the other services offered by a home health agency.

There are, of course, some audit tools available; however, all have limitations. They either restrict themselves solely to an assessment of nursing or, if they have the capacity to appraise several services, their criteria are broad and not well

Reprinted with permission from *Nursing Outlook*, 25 (March 1977), copyright © 1977, American Journal of Nursing Company, pp. 168-171.

defined. Without an operational definition of quality, or agreement about what constitutes "goodness" for each criterion of care, reviewers' judgments are guided by how they themselves would have given the care.

One possible solution to this problem is a method of quality assurance in the form of a patient care program that have been developed by our visiting nurse association and has now been in operation for 18 months.

CHARACTERISTICS OF SYSTEM

The purpose of the review program is to provide a mechanism that will enable a systematic evaluation of the quality of patient care provided to individuals in their homes, in relation to (1) patients' needs due to illness or disability, and (2) the program objectives of the agency. The ultimate objective of the review system is to improve the quality of care by assisting the agency to provide a range of home health services at optimum standards. The review program's main characteristics are:

- It is a systematic appraisal of all home health services rendered by the agency, as documented in patients' records according to the extent to which these services measure up to the operational definition of quality care. This definition is derived from the standards of care as stated in the written policies of the agency.

- It has the capacity to assess the care provided by six disciplines—nursing, home health aide, social work, and physical, speech, and occupational therapy services.

- It is accomplished through the review of a statistically valid sample of active and discharged patients' records on a bimonthly basis to determine the extent to which 28 explicit care criteria have been met.

- It focuses on overall agency performance and measures those aspects of care considered essential in providing an integrated home health service of high quality. The degree of clinical competence of individual staff personnel is not directly evaluated; instead, an indirect assessment of staff performance emerges as a by-product of the review process.

- Finally, in these days of demands for accountability, the system is a tool to answer the question: "Does a patient receive good care?"

HOW THE SYSTEM WORKS

The process of record review is carried out by a group known as the Patient Care Review Committee, consisting of four experienced staff nurses, an administrator, and one nursing supervisor. During every review sequence, each committee member audits six or seven patient records. (No member is assigned a record of a patient in whose care she has participated.) The individual reviewers then present the findings of each record assessed to the total review committee for a final determination of the quality of service rendered, as well as for decisions regarding recommendations for follow-up.

A review form is completed for each record selected for audit. The form is divided into five sections designed to assess three dimensions of care: admission to service, delivery of service, and discharge from service. The first section, Identifying Data, is completed by a clerk and consists of basic information such as diagnosis, length of service, referral source, types and volume of services, and patient status, either active or discharged, at the time of review.

The next three sections are completed by the individual reviewers. The heart of the review is the second section, Delivery of Services, which consists of the largest number of items to be evaluated—such items as the care plan, visit schedule, physician orders, medication list, and the patient profile. Criteria for each item are described and defined in the instruction sheet, and the assessment is made on the basis of actual evidence in a patient's record that the criterion has been met. Thus, for "visit schedule," the description reads as follows:

> As long as service is provided, the record shows that the visit frequency was safe and appropriate and that action plans were carried out as needed during each visit. Visit frequency should be consistent with MD orders and patient/family needs and should reflect any changes thereof. Long periods between visits (e.g., more than two weeks) which do not seem appropriate to the patient's condition should be explained in the narrative clearly (e.g., patient cancelled visit).

All reviewers, as well as the rest of the staff, have a copy of these criteria.

Each item on the review form is followed by spaces in which the reviewer checks "yes," "no," "uncertain," or "not applicable," according to whether or not the criterion has been met. "No" and "uncertain" answers must be explained in the space provided under "comments." The form for this section appears in Figure 1 and includes titles of items to be audited.

The same procedure is followed for the items listed in the third section, Discharge from Service, which is concerned with the reason for discharge and the patient's status on discharge, plans for discharge, and timeliness of the decision. In the fourth section, the Primary Reviewer's Summary, the reviewer summarizes the findings by entering the total number of criteria judged to be "yes," "no," "uncertain," "not applicable." In addition, the reviewer lists each item number that received a score of no or uncertain and the reason for the score.

FIGURE 1
Section II of the Five-Section Audit Form

AUDIT SECTION II – DELIVERY OF SERVICES

	Yes	No	Unc.	N/A	Comments
12. M.D. Orders					
13. Medication List					
14. Housing					
15. Availability of Family/Friends					
16. Care Plan A. Medical Supervision					
B. Health Needs/Action Plan					
C. Referrals					
D. Safety					
E. Goals					
17. Patient Profile					
18. Communication with M.D.					
19. Visit Schedule					
20. Service Record					
21. Ongoing Care Plan A. Periodic Patient Assessment					
B. Periodic Alteration of Care Plan					
22. Involvement of Patient/Family					
23. Non-Nursing V.N.A. Services A. M.D. Orders					
B. P.T.					
C. H.H.A.					
D. H.H.A. Supervision					
E. Social Work					
24. Communication Between Nursing & P.T.					
Summary Admission to Service Enter Total Each Column					

The patient's record and reviewer's audit form then go to the total committee whose task is to judge the quality of the care on a four-point scale from excellent (A) to poor (D). Guidelines defining criteria for each score are also included in the policy manual. For example, a score of excellent means no major defects were found or no more than two minor defects; for this score, no deficiencies can be present in the items identified as the care plan, visit schedule, ongoing care plan, physician orders, or any item under discharge from service.

Appropriate comments for the reasons for the scores are also recorded, as well as the committee's recommendation for follow-up actions, if indicated. These recommendations may be directed to the services being provided, agency policy, or coordination between community agencies, for instance. If some action is recommended, the committee specifies to whom the recommendation should be referred.

Following each record review sequence, a random sample of records rated excellent, good, fair, and poor by the review committee are reaudited and judged a second time by an impartial nurse. This monitoring mechanism assures accuracy and uniformity during the individual assessments by each reviewer as well as during the final deliberations of the review committe, in order to minimize the possibility of reviewer bias.

TESTING AND REVISION

During the testing phase of the system, the review form had 47 criteria to be assessed in the two main sections—delivery of care and discharge. After six months of use, the form was revised and the number of criteria reduced to 28. Some criteria were deleted because: (1) they were found to be purely mechanical indicators that evaluated the degree of adherence to the agency's record system, rather than the quality of services provided; (2) a few items never showed a deficiency; therefore, it was pointless as well as time consuming to continue assessing these items; and (3) two criteria dealt with team nursing, which no longer was practiced at our VNA; we had changed to district assignments. In some other instances, a few criteria were combined.

The revision of the form had two positive effects. First, it emphasized a more in-depth examination of the actual delivery of service and, second, the total time needed to complete the review form was reduced significantly, leading to a more effective, efficient patient care assessment tool.

The findings of each bimonthly review sequence are disseminated to all levels of agency personnel. For instance, each record requiring corrective action is returned to a supervisor who, in turn, discusses the review findings and the need for follow-up with the appropriate staff members. Once the corrective action has been taken, the supervisor responsible for monitoring the management of patient care notifies the review committee that the recommendations have been implemented.

Also following each review sequence, a written summary of all of the findings and recommendations is distributed to each service unit. Besides direct, formal feedback, periodic discussions concerning the findings and recommendations are held during administrative-supervisory meetings.

BUILT-IN BONUSES

This patient care review program has generated much new and worthwhile information. For the first time, hard data exist to document the quality of care provided by the agency. Also, statistics have been gathered concerning the average length of service required by certain types of patients and the volume and mix of personnel needed to provide appropriate care for each patient.

The program has also helped to identify agency strengths and weaknesses. Among the strengths identified were: responses to requests for service were promptly handled, physician orders were current and adequately executed, informal record reviews were done on schedule, on-site supervision of home health aides occurred regularly, and the skills of licensed practical nurses were appropriately utilized. A common thread ran through all of the identified strengths—that is, each strength could be classified as functional, or task-oriented.

WEAKNESS IDENTIFIED

The weaknesses that were uncovered ranged from too casual recording practices to inadequate development and execution of care plans. These too, had a common trait; all weaknesses were in the knowledge-judgment area. For instance, some common deficiencies were incomplete listing of health needs and action plans as well as sketchy patient profiles, especially in the areas of secondary diagnoses and past health history. Other weaknesses were lack of involvement of family members in patients' care, timeliness of discharge, and adequacy of discharge planning. For instance, a patient would have been discharged to a hospital or nursing home but no evidence was found in the record to indicate that pertinent health or social data were relayed by the staff member responsible for the patient's care to the facility by phone or written summary.

To reduce the incidence of deficiencies and thus improve the quality of care, various kinds of remedial programs were undertaken. For example, staff education sessions were held to improve recording techniques, to increase knowledge concerning certain disease processes, and to develop skills in assessment and comprehensive care planning. In addition, changes were made in the agency's record system, and greater emphasis was placed upon adherence to established recording practices by all staff.

The test of any quality assurance program is its impact on patient care, especially its ultimate effect in dealing with the areas identified as problems or deficiencies. Recent review sequences have shown a significant improvement in the rating scores, demonstrating that the system has improved the quality of care. Furthermore, the list of common deficiencies has decreased from 13 to 3, which represents a 77 percent reduction.

Even though staff members were involved in the development of the system and inservice programs were held prior to its implementation, reaction to the process and its findings was mixed. Many staff members supported the concepts of quality assurance and accepted the fact that health professionals operate under a social mandate that expects them to be accountable for the quality of services rendered. Other staff members, however, appeared to neither accept nor support the concepts of quality assurance. Unfortunately, the system produced feelings of threat and rejection among the noncommitted individuals.

How expensive is this program? Analysis has shown that it costs $590 to complete each review sequence. At the same time, the annual cost of the system, spread across the total illness service visits (59,566) made by our six illness service disciplines, is $.058 or not quite six cents a visit. Included in the cost are all salary and fringe benefits, time consumed completing individual record reviews and review committee meetings, preparation of committee minutes and reports, as well as time spent completing follow-up on records that were returned for corrections or recommended action.

FUTURE DIRECTIONS

At present, the system is working well and does answer the question, "Does a patient receive good care?" However, a second question—one equally important for home health agencies—needs to be addressed: "What difference does agency service make to a patient?" To find out, future efforts will be focused upon adding outcome criteria to the review procedure. By so doing, the system will then become a process-outcome method of evaluation. Continuing effort will be directed toward increasing the specificity of the rating scores.

Finally, a third modification is planned which will add another dimension to the system. Now, the primary reviewers also function as the total review committee but, in the future, the members will only assess individual records and complete the review forms. The final determination of the quality of care and recommendations for follow-up will be made by a committee composed of a physician, a nurse supervisor, two staff nurses—who are also primary reviewers—an administrator, a rehabilitation therapist, and a social worker. Such committee expansion should produce a multidisciplinary approach.

The system is not a finished product, but we believe that the valuable information we have already obtained has directly helped our staff to improve patient care and to make our services more responsive to patient needs. The fact that further refinement of our tool is necessary only serves to underline a fact that we all know: the search for an instrument to measure quality of care is a long and arduous task.

ABOUT THE AUTHOR

Elizabeth Daubert, MPH, RN, is Associate Director, Visiting Nurse Association of New Haven, New Haven, Connecticut.

A Patient Classification System in Home Health Care

Marilyn D. Harris, Charlotte Santoferraro, and Susan Silva

This piece and the one that follows demonstrate efforts built on the earlier work of Daubert. Harris and her co-authors describe efforts to develop a classification scheme for home care clients, a recognized prerequisite to the initiation of any prospective or capitated payment method for home health care. Theoretically, a valid classification framework might also yield a systematic approach to defining the outcomes of home care services.

One area of methodological research in nursing recently receiving a great deal of attention involves patient classification systems. This is not surprising because these instruments are designed to respond to varying care demands in a variety of settings by assessing patient requirements for nursing care. Nurse administrators must ensure quality care that requires adequate staffing levels and an appropriate mix of staff with sophisticated skills to meet patient needs. Factors influencing this care include government regulations, economic conditions, public scrutiny, and budget constraints. A patient classification tool that provides staffing and cost data can be invaluable.

Reprinted with permission from *Nursing Economics*, 3 (September-October 1985), copyright © 1985, Anthony J. Jannetti, Inc., pp. 276-282.

PATIENT CLASSIFICATION SYSTEMS

Definition

Patient classification systems may be broadly defined as "the grouping of patients according to some observable or inferred properties or characteristics" and "quantification of these categories as a measure of the nursing effort."[1] Those activities requiring the greatest amount of nursing care are termed critical indicators of care. Patients are assigned to an appropriate care category through assessment of the critical indicators. Two types of patient classification systems, prototype (subjective) and factor evaluation (objective), currently exist and differ in their rating methods. Although the designs are differentiated as either objective or subjective, both involve subjective judgments.

In the prototype design, each category fully describes the characteristics typifying patients in the category. Each category represents greater or lesser requirements for nursing care. Patients are simultaneously rated on a variety of critical indicators. The rater's preception of the patient's characteristics are compared to those characteristics descriptive of the category. The patient is then assigned to the category most closely matching his or her characteristics.

In the factor evaluation design, the patient's characteristics are rated individually. The individual ratings are combined to indicate an overall rating that determines the category in which the patient is classified.

Community Health Setting Classification

Hardy described a patient classification system using four nursing diagnoses (alterations in skin integrity, respiratory function, mobility, and thought processes) to represent four broad categories of home care patients.[2] Although Hardy's study of 39 patients did not find any *statistical* significance among the number of visits, duration of care, and the combination of variables studied, the data did suggest that a classification system for home health patients using nursing diagnostic categories and acuity levels can effectively predict needed nursing resources. Other researchers have also noted the potential for using nursing diagnoses and/or acuity levels to determine nursing resources.[3]

Ballard and McNamara conducted a study to determine what factors were most predictive of nursing service and total agency service required by cardiac and cancer patients in home care agencies.[4]

The study design involved retrospective record reviews in nine home health agencies. Two notable findings were: (a) Use of other agency resources was negatively correlated with the number of nursing visits per day for cancer patients; and (b) the agency differences reflected the needs of the communities served and the financial and emotional commitments exhibited by these communities as well as the agencies' philosophies and focuses of care.

Sienkiewicz examined the effects of a weighted patient classification system on the quality of care rendered by community health nurses as indicated by nursing documentation of the admission visit.[5] Sienkiewicz assigned a weighted value of 2 to an admission visit allowing equal time for direct care and indirect care documentation. The study results did not support her hypothesis that admission visits to classified patients were of higher quality than those to unclassified patients.

Daubert described the Rehabilitation Potential Patient Classification System (RPPCS) as implemented in a community health agency.[6] Daubert's copyrighted method was developed as one component of a quality assurance program to evaluate patient outcomes.

Daubert's system, a formal method of measuring patient outcomes, classifies all patients admitted to an agency's illness service program (regardless of the number of diagnoses per patient or the mix of agency services received) into one of five patient groups according to each patient's rehabilitation potential.[7]

Abbreviated descriptions of Daubert's five patient groups are:

1. Group 1—Patients who will return to pre-illness level of functioning.

2. Group 2—Patients who are experiencing an acute episode of illness but have the potential for returning to pre-episodic level of functioning.

3. Group 3—Patients who will eventually function without agency services.

4. Group 4—Patients who will remain at home as long as possible with ongoing agency service.

5. Group 5—Patients will be maintained at home during the end stage of illness for as long as possible with agency service.

For each patient group, a specific ultimate objective and a separate set of subobjectives have been identified. These subobjectives apply to all six illness service components: nursing; home health aide; physical, speech, and occupational therapies; and medical social work.

Several subobjectives are common to all groups. For example, if indicated, the patient/family will demonstrate an understanding of the prescribed diet. Other are specific to the group of patients. For example, Group 5, the patient/family, will be allowed to express feelings about dying.

All patients who receive more than two visits are admitted to Daubert's system no later than the third visit. All patients who receive one or two visits for specific reasons are also admitted. For example, the patient's care can be completed in one visit.

In this RPPCS, each applicable subobjective has to be successfully accomplished to meet the ultimate objective.

Our Visiting Nurse Association (VNA) was interested in implementing outcome criteria as part of the agency's quality assurance program and as a management tool. Daubert's system could be adapted to collect outcome data at our VNA.

Outcome criteria discharge codes were initiated during FY '80. Inservice programs were held for the staff. Definitions of terms and written instructions about how to use the system were presented to all visiting staff. Professional personnel were asked to include a two-digit code on the VNA's computer form (Patient's Master Update Form) for all patients admitted to and discharged from service with a minimum of three visits.

The first digit (0-5) was used to indicate the goal on admission to service. This goal applied to the primary diagnosis on admission (see Table 1). The VNA modified Daubert's method of indicating goal attainment on discharge. The staff was asked to quantify the goal attainment. The second digit (0-4) (see Table 1) was used to indicate this level of goal attainment on discharge from service. This two-digit code appears on the Patients Discharged This Month computer report. Data are analyzed on a monthly and annual basis

TABLE 1
Classification Codes by Rehabilitation Potential on Admission and Discharge

Goal on Admission	Goal Attainment on Discharge
Group 0. Less than three visits or not admitted to care.	Group 0. Less than three visits or not admitted to care.
Group 1. Recovery (return to pre-illness level of functioning).	Group 1. Maximum—all subobjectives met.*
Group 2. Self-care (potential to return to pre-episodic level of functioning).	Group 2. Moderate—more than half of subobjectives met.
Group 3. Rehabilitation (eventually function without agency service).	Group 3. Minimum—less than half of subobjectives met.
Group 4. Maintenance (will require ongoing agency service).	Group 4. None—none of the subobjectives met.
Group 5. Terminal Care (maintained at home during end stage of illness with agency service).	

*Subobjectives refer to those defined by Daubert for each patient group.

for several reasons: (a) to determine changes in the types of care required by patients; (b) to determine potential changes in staffing patterns; (c) to assess staff educational needs—for example, an increase in Group 5 Terminal Care patients may require additional nurses to enroll in a hospice course; (d) to evaluate agency services; and (e) to monitor cost per case.

DATA ANALYSIS

The expected Outcome Goals and Goal Attainment on Discharge codes provide important information for the management team. Two examples illustrate this point:

1. Group 5 – Terminal Care.   The VNA initiated hospice services during FY '81. The agency has a collaborative working relationship with several local hospice programs. Formal training courses and in-house terminal care committee meetings were initiated in addition to the scheduled hospice team conferences. This increased staff training and concerted effort to help patients attain their goal of dying at home are reflected in the data.

Although the overall percentages of Group 5 patients decreased during FY '83, there was a steady increase in Maximum Goal Attainment from 70 percent in FY '81 to 78 percent in FY '82 and 84 percent in FY '83. There was also the resulting decrease in None Attainment from 14 percent to 6 percent to 2 percent in these same years.

2. Group 4 – Maintenance Level.   This agency works closely with our local homemaker-home health aide service to provide maintenance level care. Funding sources differ for both agencies. Based on mutually agreeable arrangements, the VNA is able to refer patients who indicate a need for maintenance level care to the homemaker agency. Data support the supervisory staff's statement that the present referral arrangement is working well for patients and both agencies. There was a 4 percent decrease in this group of patients from FY '81 to FY '82, with the number remaining constant during FY '83. These data reflect the increasing level of skilled care required by patients referred for service.

The number of patients requiring less than three visits has increased. This finding supports statements by staff and supervisors about the increasing number of patients who are admitted to service, have the required admission paper work completed, and then are discharged for varying reasons within short periods.

Daubert states that data from the RPPCS can document the agency's effectiveness for the population served. An agency can identify its success or failure rates in terms of met or unmet service goals.

This VNA had its greatest success with Group 1 patients during FYs '81-'83. During FY '82 and FY '83, the second highest success rate in terms of maximal goal attainment was with Group 5 patients. There was a 14 percent increase in patients who were able to be at home when they died during these three years.

ECONOMIC CONSIDERATIONS

VNA Findings

Our VNA's current statistical and financial data are reported by 23 major disease categories (MDCs) grouped according to the International Classification of Diseases (ICD-9) codes, such as 000-139.9 Infectious and Parasitic Diseases, and 140-239.9 Neoplasms.[8]

Data have been available through the computer service by MDC on all discharged patients on a year-to-date basis since the beginning of FY '84. Data include: (a) length of service in days by disease category, (b) discipline, (c) average number of patient visits, (d) median length of stay, (e) total cost per case, and (f) median revenue per day. This year-to-date information can be monitored regularly to observe changes in costs and length of stay by disease category.

The RPPCS was used as a management tool to collect patient outcome data for a quality assurance program. The RPPCS also helped identify costs associated with the five rehabilitation groups and compared these costs to those associated with the MDC on a cost per case basis.

Rather than initiating a systemwide computer change in FY '84 for the purpose of collecting data by RPPCS, two graduate students in nursing service administration analyzed financial, statistical, and outcome data for a sample of patients discharged by two nurses in two geographic areas during two periods in FY '84.

The 33 patients in the sample were assigned to five groups according to their rehabilitation goals. Each goal was examined separately during the study. Data were kept on all types of services received by the patients in each group and the costs associated with each service. Individual patient data were later combined into group tables.

Table 2 shows the costs, number of visits, and time associated with the MDC for the 33 patients. Table 3 describes the same information for the 1,704 patients discharged from the agency between June 1983 and October 1984 by corresponding MDC.

Although differences existed in the average length of stay, number of visits, and time per case between the sample and population, almost no difference was noted in the average cost per case between the two groups ($705 for the

TABLE 2
Costs and Time Associated With Nine Major Disease Categories in Sample of Patients Discharged Between June 1983 and March 1984

Major Disease Category	Number	Average Length of Stay (days) on VNA Service	Average Number of Visits	Average Time in Hours	Average Cost per Case
Neoplasms	5	56	22	15	$ 767
Respiratory	2	62	25	14	657
Gastrointestinal	3	21	8	7	278
Neurologic	4	55	20	13	680
Endocrine	1	115	27	30	852
Renal	2	93	48	53	1,412
Circulatory	9	43	14	12	367
Skin/Subcutaneous	3	31	12	6	389
Musculoskeletal	4	50	30	22	947
	33				
				Average cost for sample =	$ 705

TABLE 3
Costs and Time Associated With Nine Major Disease Categories for All Patients Discharged Between June 1983 and October 1984

Major Disease Category	Number	Average Length of Stay (days) on VNA Service	Average Number of Visits	Average Time in Hours	Average Cost per Case
Neoplasms	400	33	14	16	$808
Respiratory	121	34	12	9	630
Gastrointestinal	193	19	6	3	296
Neurologic	66	41	18	13	940
Endocrine	132	32	13	5	613
Renal	51	36	13	13	707
Circulatory	590	36	15	9	734
Skin/Subcutaneous	76	29	13	8	660
Musculoskeletal	75	43	18	10	913
	1,704				
				Average cost for sample =	$700

sample and $700 for all patients). The 33 patients who were discharged by two nurses were representative of the 1,704 patients discharged by all staff during a 16-month period.

The average cost per case by MDC ($705) was similar to the average cost per case by rehabilitation goal ($696) (see Table 4).

The average age of the VNA sample was 73 years, with a range of 17 to 90 years. Seventeen patients (51.1 percent) had been hospitalized prior to their admission to the VNA.

Other data analyses involved: (a) examining the time and cost per MDC (see Table 5), and (b) comparing the nursing and medical diagnoses associated with the five rehabilitation goals (see Table 6). The one nursing diagnosis common to four of the five groups was "alteration in skin integrity." Diseases of the circulatory and musculoskeletal systems were medical diagnoses common to four of the five groups.

In the VNA sample, 665 visits were made to 33 patients. The average home care client received 22 visits at a cost of $34.54 per visit, for a total of $696 per case by RPPCS and $705 by MDC. The average length of stay was 58 days. For the VNA population of 1,704 individuals discharged between June 1983 and October 1984 and having the five corresponding MDCs, the client received an average of 13 visits at a cost of $36.89 per visit for an average cost of $700 per case. The average length of stay was 33 days.

For the VNA population of 2,287 individuals (with the nine MDCs) discharged between June 1, 1983 and March 31, 1985, the home care clients received an average of 13.5 visits at a cost of $36.78 per visit, for an average cost of $731 per case. The average length of stay was 31 days.

TABLE 4
Costs Associated with Rehabilitation Potential Goals for Sample of 33 Patients

Rehabil- itation Goals	Number	Costs by Discipline						Total Costs for Cases	Average Cost per Case
		RN[a]	PT[b]	OT[c]	SP[d]	HHA[e]	MSW[f]		
1	7	$ 3,279	$ 0	$ 0	$0	$ 330	$ 0	$ 3,609	$516
2	8	3,416	1,970	35	0	1,749	215	7,385	923
3	5	3,232	200	0	0	124	129	3,685	737
4	10	4,536	960	210	0	177	0	5,883	588
5	3	1,919	120	0	0	368	0	2,407	802
Total	33	$16,382	$3,250	$245	$0	$2,748	$344	$22,969	$696

[a] Registered nurse
[b] Physical therapist
[c] Occupational therapist
[d] Speech pathologist
[e] Home health aide
[f] Medical social worker

TABLE 5
Time and Costs by Major Disease Category for Sample of 33 Patients

Major Disease Category	Time (in hours)		Costs		Average Cost per Hour
Neoplasms	RN[a]	71.24	RN	$3,704	
	MSW[b]	2.25	MSW	129	
	Total	73.49	Total	$3,833	$52.15
Respiratory	RN	19.46	RN	$ 903	
	PT[c]	2.92	PT	200	
	OT[d]	4.71	OT	210	
	Total	27.09	Total	$1,313	$48.46
Gastrointestinal	RN	18.14	RN	$ 755	
	PT	1.75	PT	80	
	Total	19.89	Total	$ 835	$41.98
Neurologic	RN	36.46	RN	$2,821	
	PT	19.40	PT	666	
	MSW	2.36	MSW	215	
	HHA[e]	19.50	HHA	263	
	Total	77.72	Total	$3,965	$51.01
Endocrine	RN	11.72	RN	$ 616	
	HHA	17.50	HHA	236	
	Total	29.62	Total	$ 852	$28.76
Renal	RN	24	RN	$1,320	
	PT	26.26	PT	750	
	HHA	55.50	HHA	754	
	Total	105.76	Total	$2,824	$26.70
Circulatory	RN	50.53	RN	$2,033	
	PT	11.98	PT	640	
	HHA	41.33	HHA	627	
	Total	103.84	Total	$3,300	$31.77
Skin/subcutaneous	RN	18.98	RN	$1,167	
	Total	18.98	Total	$1,167	$61.48
Musculoskeletal	RN	39.14	RN	$2,409	
	PT	16.34	PT	960	
	HHA	31.15	HHA	420	
	Total	86.63	Total	$3,789	$43.73

[a] Registered nurse
[b] Medical social worker
[c] Physical therapist
[d] Occupational therapist
[e] Home health aide

TABLE 6
Medical and Nursing Diagnoses Associated with Five Rehabilitation Goals for Sample of 33 Patients

Rehabilitation Goals	Medical Diagnoses	Nursing Diagnoses
1	Musculoskeletal Circulatory Skin/subcutaneous Genitourinary	Alteration in cardiac status Knowledge deficit Alteration in skin integrity Self-care deficit
2	Endocrine Musculoskeletal Circulatory Genitourinary	Alteration in fluid-electrolyte balance Decreased mobility Knowledge deficit Adjustment to illness Alteration in metabolism
3	Musculoskeletal Neoplasm Skin/subcutaneous Circulatory	Alteration in circulatory system Alteration in skin integrity Alteration in gastrointestinal function Alteration in nutritional status
4	Endocrine Circulatory Respiratory Musculoskeletal Digestive Nervous Genitoourinary	Alteration in cardiac status Alteration in skin integrity Decreased mobility Alteration in elimination Alteration in level of consciousness
5	Respiratory Neoplasm Skin/subcutaneous	Alteration in respiratory status Self-care deficit Alteration in skin integrity

For the VNA total population of 2,940 patients discharged between June 1, 1983 and March 31, 1985 and including the 23 MDCs, the home care client received an average of 13 visits at a cost of $36.78 per visit, for an average cost of $697.85 per case. The average length of stay was 32 days.

Although the 33 patients in the sample averaged more visits and had longer average lengths of stay than the VNA population, the total cost per case varied only slightly.

National Findings and Implications

On October 1, 1984, Congressman Claude Pepper released the results of a national study of the operation, reimbursement, and cost effectiveness of home care services. The report entitled "Building a Long-Term Care System:

Home Care Data and Implications" contains the results of two independent, but related, national reviews of home health and social services.[9]

The studies were conducted by the General Accounting Office (GAO) and the Pepper Aging Committee's Subcommittee on Health and Long-Term Care, with assistance from the National Association for Home Care (NAHC). Criticisms of the NAHC study included: (a) Only 673 responses to the NAHC questionnaires sent to 4,003 certified home health agencies in July 1983 were obtained, and (b) the study's statistical validity was questionable.

The average home care client in the Pepper report received 9.6 visits at a cost of $37.95 per visit for a total of $364.32 per case. The average length of stay was about 1 month.

Abt Associates, the Health Care Financing Administration (HCFA) contractor for the home health prospective payment demonstration, found that on claims from 228 home health agencies in the five Abt demonstration states between February and July 1982, the average length of stay was 78.11 days, while the average total charge per patient was $1,172.[10] The HCFA national data from the Bureau of Data Management and Statistics cited in the Abt May 1984 report show an average of 25.5 visits per patient in 1981 and an average charge per case of $918.

Home Health Line published a comparison of costs per patient and numbers of visits for the largest city voluntary home health agencies in the United States.[11] For the 12 largest VNAs, the cost per visit ranged from $30.74 to $100.79, cost per patient from $253.56 to $1,539.54, and visits per patient from 6 to 50.

Some reasons for the variations in the data are: (a) lack of standardized definitions; (b) lack of standardized data collection; (c) differing sizes of the agencies; (d) differing ages of the agencies (for example, GAO threw out agencies that had been in operation three years or less because new agencies have higher costs and lower utilization rates, while the NAHC study included new agencies); and (e) differing criteria for data used in the studies (for example, GAO threw out provider-based data because of the add-on costs, but NAHC did not.).

Some findings of these national reports were relevant for our VNA in view of proposed changes in reimbursement for home health services. Currently, home health agencies are reimbursed on a per visit basis. However, the National Home Health Agency Prospective Payment Demonstration is being conducted under the sponsorship of HCFA to test alternative methods for reimbursing services provided by Medicare-certified home health agencies. Three different prospective payment methods will be tested: (a) reimbursement rates per visit by discipline; (b) a comprehensive monthly rate paid for each month in which patients are under the care of the provider; and (c) a comprehensive rate per episode of treatment.[12]

Although only 120 agencies in ten states will voluntarily participate in this three-year study, all agency administrators must monitor the costs of providing services by multiple classification systems through their own computer systems. By determining cost per case by MDC, cost per case by rehabilitation goal, cost per day and month, cost per visit by discipline, and cost per nursing diagnosis and acuity level, administrators can decide what changes may be required to provide the needed services within revised budget contraints.

Classification data can also help determine staffing resources, discipline mix, and internal changes necessary for providing quality health-care services with less money. Several examples of internal changes are: (a) standardized flow sheets; (b) tape recorded clinical notes,[13] (c) corporate restructuring, (d) diversification, and (e) patient teaching tools to supplement professional instructions.

FUTURE PLANS

Our VNA currently uses nursing diagnoses for problem identification and charting. We plan to code existing information, rehabilitation goals (long-range goals), and acuity levels into our computer system so that financial and time data will be generated by other classification systems.

The VNA now receives monthly computer reports that identify current and year-to-date statistics for the average hours per patient and the patient's age by payer source. This information helps the management team identify those disease categories that are most costly to staff as well as the referral sources of patients most likely to require long visits.

Patient classification systems are receiving attention as alternative reimbursement methods are proposed for home care. The various systems discussed in this article will become important management tools as reimbursement methods shift away from cost per visit.

Our VNA management team is continually seeking to improve its classification system and data collection process while enhancing our quality assurance program. By collecting financial data with multiple systems, we can manage the agency more effectively and efficiently.

ABOUT THE AUTHORS

Marilyn D. Harris, MSN, RNC, CNAA, is Executive Director, Visiting Nurse Association of Eastern Montgomery County, Abington, Pennsylvania. At the time of writing, Charlotte Santoferraro, BSN, RN, and Susan Silva, BSN, RN, were graduate students, University of Pennsylvania, Philadelphia.

The primary author acknowledges the help of Clay Figard, Vice President of Delta Computer Systems, for his help in incorporating patient classification systems into the Management Information System at the Visiting Nurse Association of Eastern Montgomery County. The VNA has purchased the right to use the Rehabilitation Potential Patient Classification System as described by Elizabeth Daubert from the Visiting Nurse Association of New Haven, CT.

REFERENCES

1. P. Giovannetti, "Understanding Patient Classification Systems," *Journal of Nursing Administration*, 9(2) (1979), 4.

2. J. A. Hardy, "A Patient Classification System for Home Health Patients," *Caring* 3(8) (1984), 26-27.

3. R. Adams and P. Duchene, "Computerization of Patient Acuity and Nursing Care Planning," *Journal of Nursing Administration*, 15(4) (1985), 11-17; L. Donnelly, "Patient Classification: An Effective Management Tool," *Nursing Management*, 12(11) 1981, 42-43; S. Grant, A. Bellinger, and B. Seda, "Measuring Productivity through Patient Classifications," *Nursing Administration Quarterly*, 30 (1982), 77-83; and M. Sovie, "Managing Nursing Resources in a Constrained Environment," *Nursing Economics*, 3(2) (1985), 85-94.

4. S. Ballard and R. McNamara, "Quantifying Nursing Needs in Home Health Care," *Nursing Research*, 32 (1983), 236-241.

5. J. Sienkiewica, "Patient Classification in Community Health Nursing," *Nursing Outlook*, 32 (1984), 219-221.

6. E. Daubert, "Patient Classification and Outcome Criteria," *Nursing Outlook*, 27 (1979), 450-454.

7. *Patient Classification/Objectives System Methodology Manual* (New Haven, CT: Visiting Nurse Association of New Haven, 1980).

8. U. S. Department of Health and Human Services, *International Classification of Diseases—Clinical Modification*, Vol. 1 (PHS) Pub. No. 80-1260 (2nd ed., 9th rev.; Washington, D.C.: U. S. Government Printing Office, 1980).

9. *Pepper Report—Building a Long-Term Care System: Home Care Data and Implications* (Washington, DC: U. S. House of Representatives Select Committee on Aging, 1984).

10. K. Rak, *Home Health Line*, (1984), 262-264.

11. K. Rak, *Home Health Line*, 10 (1985), 6.

12. J. Williams, G. Gaumer, and R. Schmitz, *National Home Health Agency Prospective Payment Demonstration Project Description* (Cambridge, MA: Abt Associates, April 1985).

13. M. Harris, "A Tape Recording and Transcribing System to Maintain Patients' Clinical Records," *Nursing & Health Care*, 5 (1984), 503-507.

Relating Quality and Cost in a Home Health Care Agency

Marilyn D. Harris, Donna A. Peters, and Joan Yuan

In recent years health care providers have felt increasing pressure from consumers, third-party payers, and regulators to contain costs while maintaining or even improving quality. More than ever before, patients—especially the large and growing elderly population—are aware of health issues and of their rights as patients and consumers. Their families are similarly aware, and they are concerned about the safety and well-being of their loved ones. Medicare and other third-party payers are demanding quality and utilization review efforts to ensure that the financial incentives offered by prospective payment and other reimbursement schemes do not compromise the quality of care.

This pressure has encouraged quality assurance (QA) to shift its focus from the processes used by practitioners to the outcomes experienced by patients,[1] and has made it imperative to integrate QA and cost-containment systems. The information generated by such an integrated system allows the provider to understand quality in relation to cost and thereby to combine quality with efficiency—a combination essential for survival in the new competitive environment.[2]

Reprinted with permission from *Quality Review Bulletin,* (May 1987), copyright © 1987, Joint Commission on the Accreditation of Hospitals, pp. 175–181.

The same pressure that has brought about this new thinking in QA has made home health care an important alternative, particularly for the elderly. Like most other providers, most home health care agencies operate with a philosophy that demands quality. At the same time, like other providers, agencies must find ways to offer quality care while operating efficiently. This article describes an integrated QA-cost-containment system, based on expected outcomes for various patient categories, developed for use in a home health care agency.

The Visiting Nurse Association (VNA) of Eastern Montgomery County (Pennsylvania) is a voluntary, nonprofit, community health agency that makes approximately 58,000 home visits annually. Before the implementation of the outcome-based system, the VNA's QA program used structure and process criteria and gathered data by means of patient and physician questionnaires, untilization reviews, and quarterly, process-oriented patient record audits that focused on practitioner activities. The new system, implemented in August 1985, was designed to collect data about outcomes—measurable changes in patient health status, knowledge, compliance and satisfaction[3]— and about the costs associated with those changes.

To assure the validity and reliability of outcome data, the VNA used the Rehabilitation Potential Patient Classification System (RPPCS).[4] Upon admission, a patient is classified into one of five categories—recovery (Category 1), self-care (Category 2), rehabilitation (Category 3), maintenance (Category 4), or terminal (Category 5)—according to specific criteria. Expected outcomes (an objective and subobjectives) are specified for each categry (see Figure 1). During ongoing review and at discharge, the patient record must contain evidence that the subobjectives have been addressed; goal attainment is rated at three levels: "goal attained" (i.e., all subobjectives were met), "moderate attainment" (i.e., some but not all subobjectives were met), and "goal not attained" (i.e., no subobjectives were met). For each category, there is a specific documentation format, including preprinted general assessment and discharge summary sheets that list the applicable objective and subobjectives (see Figs. 2 and 3). Tools used for record reviews are likewise category-specific.

Within each category, as well as independent of category, important nursing diagnoses have been identified. To date, standardized flow sheets have also been developed for 15 of these most common nursing diagnoses (see Fig. 4). These sheets increase the efficiency of documentation, help in identifying the parameters of quality care for specific diagnoses, and aid in gathering cost data, since nursing diagnoses have a greater influence than medical diagnoses on the level of care, frequency and length of visits, and overall duration of services in a home health care setting.

On a discharge summary form, the nurse estimates the time devoted to each of the patient's nursing diagnoses as a percentage of total time spent with the patient. The total cost of nursing care is then divided by the time

FIGURE 1
Patient Classifications and Outcome Objectives Used in the Quality Assurance Program at the Visiting Nurse Association of Eastern Montgomery County

PATIENT CLASSIFICATION/OBJECTIVE SYSTEM[a]

Patient Group I (Recovery)

Patient with acute episodic-type disease or disabilty (e.g., wound infection, fracture, pneumonia, poor nutritional habits, gastrointestinal disorder, uncomplicated surgical procedure, gestational diabetes, gestational hypertension) who will return to pre-illness level of functioning. Patients in Group I should not have a primary or secondary diagnosis of chronic disease (e.g., cancer, arthritis, chronic obstructive pulmonary disease, cerebrovascular accident, heart disease, peripheral vascular disease, renal disease, hypertension, diabetes).

1. *Ultimate Program Objective for Group I*
   Patient will achieve complete recovery from illness, or patient's immediate health need/problem, which prompted admission to service (e.g., need to learn proper use of crutches or walker, need to learn correct technique for dressing change), will be eliminated.

2. *Program Subobjectives for Group I*
   a. Patient/family will demonstrate ability to assume responsibility for any ongoing medical supervision.
   b. If indicated, patient/family will demonstrate understanding of prescribed diet.
   c. If indicated, patient/family will demonstrate understanding of prescribed medication regimen.
   d. If indicated, patient/family will demonstrate ability to independently perform prescribed treatments/exercises.
   e. If indicated, patient/family will demonstrate knowledge of important safety measures.

Patient Group II (Self-Care)

Patients with early stage chronic diseases or disabilities who are experiencing an acute episode of illness but have the potential for returning to pre-episodic level of functioning (e.g., patients with cardiac disease, diabetes, cerebrovascular accident, with no residual or sight hemiparesis, chronic obstructive pulmonary disease, arthritis, hypertension).

1. *Ultimate Program Objective for Group II*
   Patient/family will manage chronic health problems without ongoing visiting nurse services.

2. *Program Subobjectives for Group II*
   a. Patient/family will demonstrate ability to assume responsibility for maintaining ongoing medical supervision.
   b. If indicated, patient/family will demonstrate understanding of prescribed diet.
   c. If indicated, patient/family will demonstrate understanding of prescribed medication regimen.
   d. If indicated, patient/family will demonstrate ability to independently perform prescribed treatments/exercises.
   e. Patient/family will recognize signs of significant physical or emotional changes as well as the need to communicate these changes to the appropriate health care provider.
   f. If indicated, patient/family will demonstrate understanding of restrictions imposed by the illness or disability.
   g. If indicated, patient/family will demonstrate knowledge of important safety measures.

Patient Group III (Rehabilitation)

Patients with
   a. intermediate stage chronic diseases or disabilities for whom a return to pre-illness level of functioning is not possible, but who have the potential for increasing level of functioning and who will eventually function without visiting nurse services, or
   b. advanced stage chronic diseases or disabilities who do not have the potential for increasing level of functioning but who, with assistance from family members, will eventually function without visiting nurse services.

FIG. 1 (continued)

Examples include patients with cardiac diseases, cerebrovascular/accident with hemiparesis, arthritis, congestive heart failure, amputated limb, blindness, and diabetes.

1. *Ultimate Program Objective for Group III*
   Patient will be rehabilitated to maximum level of physical, emotional, and social functioning, and patient/family will manage chronic health problems without continued visiting nurse services.

2. *Program Subobjectives for Group III*
   a. Patient/family will demonstrate ability to assume responsibility for maintaining ongoing medical supervision.
   b. If indicated, patient/family will demonstrate understanding of prescribed diet.
   c. If indicated, patient/family will demonstrate understanding of prescribed medication regimen.
   d. If indicated, patient/family will demonstrate ability to independently perform prescribed treatments/exercises.
   e. Patient/family will demonstrate ability to recognize signs of significant physical or emotional change as well as the need to communicate these changes to the appropriate health care provider.
   f. If indicated, patient/family will demonstrate understanding of restrictions imposed by the patient's illness.
   g. If indicated, patient/family will demonstrate knowledge of important safety measures.

Patient Group IV (Maintenance)

Patients with advanced stage chronic diseases or disabilities who can be maintained at home only with ongoing visiting nurse services. Examples include patients with advanced heart disease, neurological problems, severe arthritis, organic brain syndrome, fractures, gastrointestinal disorder, cerebrovascular accident with residual hemiplegia, cancer, and pernicious anemia.

1. *Ultimate Program Objective for Group IV*
   Patient will be maintained at home as long as possible with ongoing visiting nurse services.

2. *Program Subobjectives for Group IV*
   a. Patient/family will demonstrate ability to assume responsibility for maintaining ongoing medical supervision.
   b. If indicated, patient/family will demonstrate understanding of prescribed diet.
   c. If indicated, patient/family will demonstrate understanding of prescribed medication regimen.
   d. If indicated, patient/family will demonstrate ability to perform prescribed treatments/exercises.
   e. Patient/family will demonstrate ability to recognize significant physical or emotional change as well as the need to communicate these changes to the appropriate health care provider.
   f. If indicated, patient/family will demonstrate understanding of restrictions imposed by the patient's illness.
   g. If indicated, patient/family will demonstrate knowledge of important safety measures.

Patient Group V (Terminal)

Patients with an end-stage illness, such as terminal chronic obstructive pulmonary disease, cancer, renal failure, cardiac disease, cirrhosis.

1. *Ultimate Program Objective for Group V.*
   Patient will be maintained at home during the end stage of illness as long as possible with visiting nurse services.

2. *Program Subobjectives for Group V*
   a. Patient/family will demonstrate ability to assume responsibility for maintaining ongoing medical supervision.
   b. If indicated, patient/family will demonstrate understanding of prescribed diet.
   c. If indicated, patient/family will demonstrate understanding of prescribed medication regimen.
   d. If indicated, patient/family will demonstrate ability to perform prescribed treatments/exercises.
   e. Patient/family will demonstrate ability to recognize signs of significant physical or emotional change as well as the need to communicate these changes to the appropriate health care provider.
   f. Patient/family will receive emotional support as needed.

FIG. 1 (continued)

g. Patient/family will be allowed to express feelings about dying.
h. Patient/family will receive assistance as needed to prepare for death.
i. If indicated, patient/family will demonstrate knowledge of important safety measures.

---

[a] Adapted from The Visiting Nurse Association of New Haven Patient Classification/Objective System

devoted to each nursing diagnosis. Monthly computer-generated reports (see Fig. 5) give statistical and financial data, including volume, frequency of visits, overall duration of whose services, and costs for each nursing diagnosis and patient category. Other computer reports also display goal attainment levels.

Such information can be used to answer a variety of questions from the point of view of quality and efficiency. For example, in the case of a patient whose duration of services was longer than average, was the longer stay essential to quality? Was care of comparable quality given to similar patients who had shorter stays? If so, what patient characteristics or aspects of care distinguished these patients? Did the longer stay result from agency policy? If so, is that policy appropriate? Could the needs of the longer-staying patient have been met more efficiently, as with a special program or specially trained staff? If not, should patients of this type be admitted to service?

Over time, such information can lead to the identification of patterns that may need to be addressed. For example, certain problem diagnoses may be found to be associated with each other, or certain problems may be traceable to a particular referral source that should be notified (e.g., if many patients from a single institution need care for wound infections, the agency may be able to help the referral institution identify an infection control problem).

One interesting phenomenon discovered at the VNA is that patients who are cost-outliers with regard to the nursing diagnosis of "self-care deficit" are often also cost-outliers with regard to other nursing diagnoses. For example, Ms. P, an 86-year-old woman in Category 3 who lived with her legally blind son, was identified as a cost-outlier with regard to the diagnoses of "self-care deficit" and "actual alteration in skin integrity." Her medical condition included a venous stasis ulcer of the right lower extremity, a pressure sore of the sacrum, diabetes, arteriosclerotic cardiovascular disease, chronic obstructive pulmonary disease, urinary tract infection, and lymphoma. Her nursing diagnoses included "actual impairment of skin integrity," "self-care deficit," "alteration in urinary elimination," and "alteration in health maintenance." These nursing problems were resolved, with 60 percent of the nurses' time devoted to actual impairment of skin integrity ($2,214.50), 25 percent to self-care deficit ($922.50), 10 percent to alteration in urinary elimination ($369.00), and 5 percent to alteration in health maintenance ($184.50). Review verified the correctness of Ms. P's categorization and nurs-

FIGURE 2
Example of Patient-Category-Specific General Assessment Format

FLOW SHEET
GENERAL ASSESSMENT V
END STAGE: TERMINAL CARE

PT. # _____   NAME _____   PG. _____   DATE OF VISIT 19 _____

DATE	PROB. #	PARAMETERS/ INTERVENTIONS		FREQ.
		VITAL SIGNS	B.P.	
			P.	
			R/T	
		BREATH SOUNDS	RUL	
			RML	
			RLL	
			LUL	
			LLL	
		Assess Edema - Pedal Rt/Lt		
		Assess Learning Ability		
		Assess Nutritional Status/Appetite		
		Diet Instruction		
		Demonstrates Understanding of Diet		
		Evaluate Elimination Patterns		
		Assess/Instruct Medication Regimen		
		Demonstrates Understanding of Meds		
		Assess Ability to Perform Treatments		
		Treatment Instruction		
		Demonstrates Ability to do Treatments		
		Assess/Instruct Safety in Home		
		Demonstrates Knowledge of Safety Measures		
		Next M.D. Visit		
		Pt.Recognizes Physical/Emotional Changes		
		Communicates Chgs.to Approp. Professional		
		Assess Emotional Status/Coping Mechanisms		
		Allow Expression Re: Dying		
		Provide Emotional Support		
		Assist as Necessary in Preparation of Death.		

CODE BREATH SOUNDS
1 FULL
2 DIMINISHED
3 ABSENT

CODE ADVENTITIOUS SOUNDS
0 NONE
1 RALES
2 RONCHI
3 WHEEZES
4 FRICTION RUB

NEXT VISIT
BILLING
INITIALS

INIT.	SIGNATURE	INIT.	SIGNATURE	INIT.	SIGNATURE	INIT.	SIGNATURE

CODES

C	Care	N	Narrative	S	Supervision
D	Discussion	NA	Not Assessed	U	Unchanged
DNA	Does Not Apply	IB	Instruction Begun	+	Yes
E	Evaluation	IC	Instruction Continued	-	No

FIGURE 3
Example of Patient-Category-Specific Discharge Summary Format

---

Discharge Summary, Patient Category V
End Stage: Terminal Care

Name _____ Patient # _____ Date _____

Ultimate Objective: Patient will be maintained at home during the end stage of illness for as long as possible with VNA services.

Nursing Action   **Patient Outcome**

Subobjectives	Assessment	Instruction	Demonstration of Increased Knowledge, Understanding, or Behavioral Change
Diet			
Medication regimen			
Treatments			
Safety measures			
Medical supervision			
Recognizes physical/ emotional change			
Communicates change to appropriate professional			
Emotional support/ coping mechanisms			
Expressed feelings about dying			
Received assistance to prepare for death			

Goal attainment is determined by demonstrating that applicable subobjectives were met/nursing problems resolved.

Action must be taken and patient/family must demonstrate increased knowledge, understanding, and/or behavioral change as a result of nurse's intervention.

Goal Attainment Code: _____#1 Maximum All applicable subobjectives were met/ nursing problems resolved.
 _____#2 Moderate Less than 100% of total goal attainment.
 _____#3 None None of the applicable subobjectives were met/ nursing problems resolved.

Summary of Services _____

_____

Problems:
#101 O/A _____

_____

#102 O/A _____

_____

#103 O/A _____

_____

#104 O/A _____

_____

© VNA of EMC 1985   Signature _____

FIGURE 4
Example of Nursing-Diagnosis Flow Sheet for the Diagnosis of Ineffectual Breathing Pattern

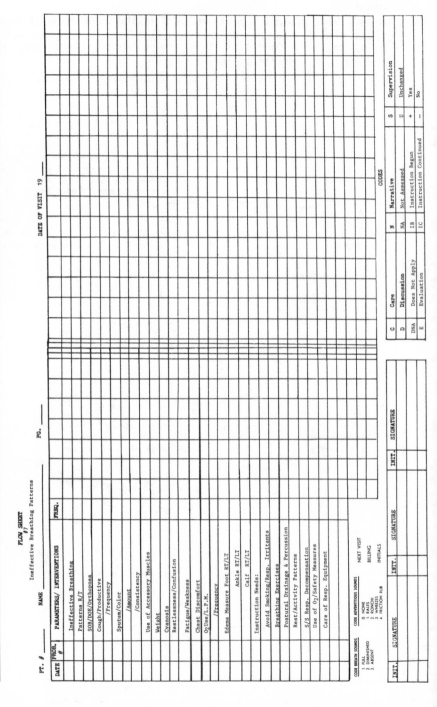

FIGURE 5

Sample Monthly Computer Report That Gives Statistical and Financial Data Associated with the Nursing Diagnoses for those Patients in Goal 3 (Rehabilitation Classification) that have Diseases of the Circulatory System

VISITING NURSE ASSOCIATION OF EASTERN MONTGOMERY COUNTY

Nursing Diagnosis　　　　　　Nursing Diagnosis Statistics by Illness Within Goal

Rehabilitation Diseases of
Circulatory System

	Number in Group	Average Time	Average Case Charge	Average Visits	Average Stay
Activity intolerance					
Ineffective airway clearance	1	4	225	10	37
Anxiety					
Alteration in bowel elimination: constipation	8	2	124	8	29
Alteration in bowel elimination: diarrhea	1	1	56	5	17
Alteration in bowel elimination: incontinence	1	1	41	7	20
Ineffective breathing patterns	46	4	291	11	38
Alteration in cardiac output: decreased	5	5	351	12	50
Alteration in comfort: pain	4	1	55	6	35
Impaired verbal communication					
Ineffective individual coping	4	3	173	11	37
Ineffective family coping: compromised					
Ineffective family coping: disabling					
Family coping: potential for growth					
Diversional activity deficit					
Alteration in family processes					
Fear					
Fluid volume deficit					
Potential fluid volume deficit					
Excess fluid volume					
Impaired gas exchange					
Anticipatory grieving					
Dysfunctional grieving					
Alteration in health maintenance	410	5	310	8	31
Impaired home maintenance management	15	4	253	8	28
Potential for injury	3	4	252	12	46
Knowledge deficit	48	3	183	9	32
Impaired physical mobility	36	3	184	7	34
Noncompliance	1	1	61	9	22
Alteration in nutrition: less than body requirements	3	4	279	13	77
Alteration in nutrition: more than body requirements	1	1	72	4	10
Alteration in nutrition: potential more than body requirements					
Alteration in oral mucous membrane					
Alteration in parenting					
Potential alteration in parenting					
Powerlessness					
Rape-trauma syndrome	2	1	53	6	19
Self-care deficit	112	2	98	9	40
Self-esteem disturbance					
Sensory-perceptual alterations					

FIG. 5 (continued)

Sexual dysfunction					
Actual impairment of skin integrity	41	3	219	10	33
Potential impairment of skin integrity	2	5	342	17	60
Disturbance in sleep pattern					
Social isolation					
Spiritual distress					
Alteration in thought processes	8	2	130	7	25
Alteration in tissue perfusion	13	3	188	7	25
Alteration in pattern of urinary					
elimination	11	3	151	10	33
Potential for violence					

ing diagnoses, the quality of her care, and the appropriate utilization of services in her care. All subobjectives for Category 3 were met. Her care was costly, however, because of its duration and complexity.

In any health care organization, the QA program has several important functions, including evaluating and improving the quality of care, meeting the standards of accrediting and regulatory bodies, managing risk, and so on. In today's increasingly consumer-minded and competitive health care environment, it is also important for the QA program to be able to relate quality to cost. As this article has shown in the case of a home health care agency, such an integrated system can be established using patient outcome criteria as a guide for measuring quality and costs.

ABOUT THE AUTHORS

Marilyn D. Harris, MSN, RNC, CNAA, is Executive Director, Visiting Nurse Association of Eastern Montgomery County, Abington, Pennsylvania. Donna A. Peters, MA, RN, CNAA, is Director of Nursing Research and Quality Assurance, The Johns Hopkins Hospital, Baltimore, Maryland. Joan Yuan, MSN, RNC, is Supervisor for Quality Assurance Program, Visiting Nurse Association of Eastern Montgomery County.

REFERENCES

1. K. Martin and N. Sheet, "The Omaha System: Implications for Costing Community Health Nursing," in F. A. Shaffer, ed., *Costing Out Nursing: Pricing Our Product* (New York: National League for Nursing, 1985), pp. 197–206.

2. C. G. Meisenheimer, *Quality Assurance: A Complete Guide to Effective Programs* (Rockville, MD: Aspen, 1985).

3. J. C. Schmadl, "Quality Assurance: Examination of the Concept," *Nursing Outlook,* 27 (July 1979), 463.

4. E. Daubert, "Patient Classification Systems and Outcome Criteria," *Nursing Outlook,* 27 (July 1979), 450–454.